Learning Psychotherapy

Learning Psychotherapy

RATIONALE AND GROUND RULES

HILDE BRUCH, M.D.

Harvard
University
Press

*Cambridge
Massachusetts
London
England*

Library of Congress Catalog Card Number 74-83848
ISBN 0-674-52025-4 (cloth)
ISBN 0-674-52026-2 (paper)

To the memory of my teachers

Frieda Fromm-Reichmann 1889–1957
Harry Stack Sullivan 1892–1949
Lawrence S. Kubie 1896–1973

Preface

The process of learning psychotherapy is lifelong: an interminable task of creative reappraisal, of studying both failures and successes with the same objectivity and readiness to learn. A therapist cannot increase his professional expertise through repetition of what he has done or been taught before. Each new patient must be approached as what he is, a stranger whose anguish and problems are unprecedented and unique; the challenge is to approach him in a special way, geared to his particular situation. This very alertness to the newness of each therapeutic encounter permits the mature therapist to use past experience as well as present ignorance in a constructive way.

These advanced achievements of psychotherapy may be a faraway goal, but it is one that needs to be implied in the learning process from the very beginning. This book addresses itself to the beginner who is for the first time confronted with the task of functioning as a psychotherapist. Learning psychotherapy is the core, the very heart, of the psychiatric residency. Over the past few decades the field of psychiatry has broadened considerably, encompassing a variety of new tasks which are usually ill defined and demand different, often contradictory, approaches and attitudes. Even with all these changes, becoming an effective psychotherapist has retained a central position. It is the only way residents can learn in depth about the complexity of human beings; such knowledge can then be applied to other treatment modalities, not only in intensive dynamic therapy.

Psychotherapy itself is in such a state of flux, and the concept has been broadened to such an extent, that nearly every professional interaction between two people, or groups of people, is referred to as "therapy." Psychoanalysis and its offspring, dynamic psychotherapy, have come under attack as being too time-consuming and expensive, and not suitable for all patients; the one-to-one relationship has been criticized as representing an outmoded "medical model" of psychiatry, out of step with modern concepts of a "social model." Most of these criticisms reflect a lack of understanding and knowledge of the essential tasks of intensive psychotherapy.

It is correct that dynamic psychotherapy makes great demands on therapist and patient alike, not only in the expenditure of time and money but in the intensity of personal involvement, in the need for introspection and willingness to be unsparingly honest and to face unpleasant facts. It demands the readiness to reexamine one's motives and attitudes toward life, and to use this understanding responsibly to take new action. That this treatment is not readily available, or even suitable, for the many does not make it less valuable or indispensable for those who can and do benefit from it, for those who find it the only way of obtaining lasting relief from their self-doubt and sorrow. Undoubtedly, many people in quandaries can benefit from some of the current streamlined, get-well-quickly approaches. Yet there are many others who require deeper self-understanding and stimulation for genuine inner growth, and they can achieve this only through individual psychotherapy. The tragic fate of patients who are reduced to powerlessness in the depersonalized setting of psychiatric hospitals that use only standard prescription of the treatment in vogue, with no relevance to the individual's needs, has been noted over the ages.

Preface

Psychotherapy addresses itself to the inner difficulties that interfere with an individual's ability to cope with the tasks and stresses inherent in human life. Students often ask what psychotherapy really is, and how it accomplishes favorable change, particularly when the available time is limited. I should like to define it here as a situation where two people interact and try to come to an understanding of one another, with the specific goal of accomplishing something beneficial for the complaining person. Though patients come to psychiatrists with a multitude of problems, I shall consider their difficulties here, in a gross oversimplification, under the heading of one common problem: the sense of helplessness, the fear and inner conviction of being unable to "cope" and to change things. This feeling can be recognized as an essential issue in every situation, though in widely varying degrees. Patients often expect, and so do beginner psychotherapists, that psychotherapy will solve their problems and make them happy, or at least less dissatisfied. If this occurs, it is a fortunate side effect. It is not in our power to make people happy, but we can be of assistance in making them at least to some degree more competent in evaluating realistically what troubles them so that they can learn to react appropriately to their problems and find relief from their sense of impotence.

And how is this achieved? In every form of psychotherapy several processes go on simultaneously and serially: by *listening* effectively to what the patient has to say, you may make him feel he has been heard and understood; by summarizing and *reformulating* what you have heard, you may help him take the first steps toward clarifying and reducing the underlying confusion that complicates his life; finally, by a more objective assessment of his resources and by *presenting alternatives,* you may help him arrive at a point where he can take action, no longer so helplessly caught in his anxieties and victimized by circumstances. These are the essential tasks of both short-term

and long-term therapy, in whatever elaborate form it is practiced. Treatment itself is the process through which a patient
develops new mental tools so that he can manage his life in a
more realistic way, less distorted, less burdened by misinterpretations and repressed emotions.

I shall attempt here to review what I have observed while
supervising the first efforts at psychotherapy of medical students,
psychiatric residents, social workers, and interns in psychology,
and also the work of candidates in psychoanalytic training who
already had extensive experience. Much was learned from my
work as consultant to practicing psychiatrists who asked for an
evaluation of patients who seemed to be untreatable. In spite of
the widely different level of expertness, there have been amazing
similarities in basic problems that were recognized as interfering
with therapeutic effectiveness. The difficulties usually rested in
preconceived notions and convictions, gleaned from previous
teaching or reading, that were not appropriate for a particular
patient and interfered with the therapist's open-minded assessment of the treatment needs.

Most of the examples used to illustrate various points have
been taken from the records of patients treated by residents,
including some from my own residency. Though they were
chosen as presenting typical problems, no generalized deductions
should be made from them when dealing with another patient;
in spite of apparent similarity, there is always need for individual modification. Psychodynamic understanding implies an
approach to the underlying problems of each person appropriate
for his particular development and needs. Only in this way will
therapy be effective and reality-oriented. Such individualization
is also an important aspect of the learning process. Each therapist needs to develop his assets and abilities in a way that is
meaningful to him. With the development of more sensitive and
deeper self-understanding he will learn to use the human rela-

tionship in an individualistic but still planned and disciplined way.

One great difficulty in the process of learning is the fact that theoretical principles and so-called techniques are often transmitted and received through stereotyped tradition-bound instruction. Probably each experienced therapist has developed a working theory and method of his own, what he actually does in the privacy of his office. However, the way he uses these personal concepts in his work with patients usually goes unstated, and what gets into print are variations on the officially accepted theories, expressed in standardized terminology. So I shall attempt a more direct personal approach here: to give some general principles underlying effective psychotherapy, within a broad theoretical frame, and to spell out some of the actual factors that help or hinder the beginner in the process of learning psychotherapy.

Contents

Contents

Learning Psychotherapy

1

When Strangers Meet

"A journey of a thousand miles begins with but a single step."
This old Chinese proverb may well be applied to the psychotherapeutic journey. However long it takes and no matter how
involved it becomes, it does begin with the initial interview;
what is experienced then and there may well determine the
course of therapy. It may start auspiciously, with a promise of
mutual rapport and understanding. Though many difficulties will
arise as treatment progresses, this basic feeling of having been
understood may well sustain the patient when the going gets
rough. Just as in a physical journey when the inattentive and
doubting may stumble and then limp along hesitatingly and with
distress, so it may happen that there are misunderstandings in
the initial contact, no reassurance to the patient that the therapist has grasped what troubles him. Unexpressed doubts and
anxieties will interfere with the therapeutic process and slow
things down. If things miscarry altogether, the trip is off; the
patient will not return. If he cannot avoid it, as when he is
hospitalized, he will remain hostile, suspicious, and uncommunicative. Such negativism is not always due to poor motivation or
paranoic attitudes of a patient, but not uncommonly it is related
to some unfortunate experience on first contact, where he might
have felt that he was dealt with as "a case" or that the therapist

did not respect him and appreciate his problems as those of a suffering human being.

The beginner is in an unusually difficult position. When a psychiatrist is established in his own practice, or has a position of prestige and authority in an institution, patients are specifically referred to him, usually with some words of praise about his special abilities. In contrast, the beginner is an unknown quantity, and a patient's reaction and the development of trust in him as a therapist are much more dependent on what he experiences in the first treatment session. Fortunately, though, in his need and desire for help a patient is ready to endow the future therapist with special competence and ability for understanding.

FIRST REACTIONS

Both the therapist and patient bring their own personalities and past experiences to the therapeutic encounter, although the therapist, let us hope, has some greater awareness of the hidden factors and fewer anxieties about what lies ahead. Whatever the overt reason and manifest symptomatology that bring a patient into a psychiatrist's office, the therapist must be motivated by the wish to be of use to the patient and to understand him, and to give him the opportunity to express himself openly and freely. Whatever he has heard about his patient-to-be, or read in the sometimes voluminous case history, when the first interview finally takes place he does well to remember that this is an occasion where two strangers meet, with both having to take the first tentative steps to learn to know one another. It is a time of mutual assessment, though there may be only limited awareness of the interplay of many subtle emotional factors. How the initial interview turns out depends on the patient and his problems, how he presents himself, how he perceives or misperceives the situation, but also on the therapist's open-mindedness, his awareness of himself and his feelings and reactions, his confidence in what he is doing, and his sensitivity to the patient's need for help and understanding.

The official task of the first interview is to get acquainted, to obtain a brief history of the patient's problems and difficulties, to form a tentative diagnostic impression, and to give some kind of formulation of the basic issues and possible treatment goals. It would be presumptuous to pretend to gain a clear, let alone complete, picture of a patient's difficulties. But it is helpful to say a few summarizing words about what one thinks the bewilderment or apprehension or anger is about. I find it useful to make some comment with a positive meaning, implying that I can conceive of the patient in a different mode, not as anxiety-ridden or depressed, suspicious, and desperate, but as a functioning person with the capacity for trust and self-confidence. A simple question might do it: "When did you last feel comfortable (or confident) about yourself?" Or one might ask a mother who has filled the whole session with a long list of her child's shortcomings and her own tribulations, "What do you enjoy most about Johnnie?"

The beginner may be too anxiously preoccupied with gathering as much information as possible and thus may focus too mechanically on getting definite answers to his many questions. In this way he may miss the all-important purpose of a first interview, namely to establish the possibility of meaningful exchange. This requires a free-flowing expression not only of words but of sentiments that convey the promise of mutual trust. Whatever the content of the discussion, another process goes on simultaneously, that of sizing one another up in terms of one's own emotional reactions. As in all important relationships, an immediate flood of feelings is aroused on first contact, which may be familiarity and liking but also remoteness or definite dislike. The alert observer will pay attention to what it is that arouses such positive or negative feelings, and whether they are fleeting or of a depth that might interfere with the development of intimacy that is a prerequisite for therapy. Feelings of liking and disliking are based on the numerous, often imponderable personal expressions and qualities that make up the total nexus of one's own background and development. An experienced therapist will disqualify himself with a face-saving explanation, without hurting the patient's feelings, and will refer him to another therapist when he notices such feelings of dislike in himself, or even when he fails to experience some sense of empathy, of potentially sympathetic understanding of the patient's problems. The beginner does not have this freedom of choice, nor the sense of definiteness about his own reactions. One way he gains experience in the training period is to learn about the range of his reactions and interactions with a great many different people. Under observation and scrutiny, he may find it difficult to admit any negative feelings in himself. As in all other relationships, it is the hidden and unacknowledged feelings that may cause trouble and interfere with the honest and open exploration of feelings and reactions as they develop in the course of therapy.

ASSESSMENT OF A STRANGER

Many of the basic issues that come up with a new patient are similar to experiences we have had throughout our lives when meeting new people and getting acquainted with them. When we meet a stranger we take in, without thinking about it, many small details about him, and we form some immediate impression of the sort of person he is, by the way he walks or dresses, his facial expression, tone of voice and gestures, eye contact or its avoidance. We automatically draw some conclusions, which may or may not be correct; we also may or may not be fully aware of them, but they find a counterexpression in our own responses, gestures, tone of voice, alertness of remarks, and so on. It is often these nonverbal messages which account for our feeling comfortable or uncomfortable when we meet a person for the first time.

If the therapist tries too hard to exclude such life-long patterns of reaction behind a stereotyped professional facade, the whole exchange may become artificial and stilted, lacking in spontaneity and warmth. An important aspect of one's development as a psychotherapist is your becoming acutely aware of the range of your own reactions and feeling tones. This reaction may also be of importance in forming a diagnostic impression. European authors continue to speak of the "praecox feeling"; on analysis this proves to be the examiner's uneasiness when the customary responses in verbal and nonverbal communication with schizophrenics do not occur. The feeling of being drained or exasperated and bewildered, which many therapists experience during conferences with the parents of schizophrenic patients, has proved an important guidepost in exploring the confusing climate and style of communication of such families.

THERAPEUTIC PURPOSE

The therapeutic interview differs from the ordinary social contact in one important respect: it is an encounter with a definite *purpose,* namely that something of positive value and constructive usefulness for the patient should come out of it. I find it useful at the outset to state this implied purpose in some explicit way, in particular if a patient finds it difficult to talk about himself. How the initial interview turns out depends, of course, on many circumstances. It will be different for a hospitalized patient who may be there against his will and who finds himself assigned to some stranger called "his therapist"; he may rebel against divulging his innermost and often frightening thoughts and feelings to this stranger. Even a patient who appears in your office on his own may find it a difficult task to confide in a complete stranger, and the neophyte therapist may ask himself, "Why should he trust me?" Direct verbal assertions—"You can tell me everything"—will disclaim by their very pompousness the subtle reassurance the patient needs and which is given in nonverbal expressions of warmth and sympathy, and by careful questions and comments that reveal a willingness to understand.

The patient is in the help-seeking role, and though he may resent the very fact of having admitted that he is not able to handle his own affairs, he usually arrives with the hope of finding support in his efforts to leave outworn patterns behind, and thus is determined to tell it all. He endows the therapist with qualities of special knowledge and authority, and this is quite independent of the age, sex, and experience of the therapist, which facilitates a patient's being open and confiding about what troubles him. Whether or not this first confession of difficulties develops into something that has the elements of a beginning therapeutic alliance depends on whether he undergoes the emotional experience of having made contact, of having found a sympathetic and understanding listener.

KEEPING THE INTERVIEW GOING

Though patients vary greatly in their readiness and ability to talk—some pour out their endless complaints without giving the listener a chance to get a word in edgewise—the more common problem is how to keep the interview going. After the first statement of what troubles him the patient expects guidance on what he should talk about, and the therapist should supply it through carefully formulated comments and questions. This is where one's *general* grasp of an individual's difficulties, and the quality of one's understanding of psychopathology, makes a great difference. Without a general familiarity with the phenomenon, one does not know what to look for and may miss the point completely. Still, rigid preconceived notions may guide one in the wrong direction and lead to irrelevant questions. I shall give a general outline of modern concepts of personality development in the next chapter.

The closer one's comments and questions relate to what the patient has expressed as troubling him, the better the interview will progress, with increasingly confidential elaborations and often a visible relief of anxiety. If on the other hand a tense beginner, perhaps with a case conference in mind, throws unconnected questionnaire-like questions at a patient, the more likely it is that the patient's tension will increase and that he will withdraw and become uncommunicative. Usually this type of questioning represents the beginner's puzzlement about what a relevant comment might be. Through attention for what one is doing, and open-minded supervision, this inexpertness gradually corrects itself with time. The process will be aided by the therapist's freedom to draw on his human resources, on his general education and the range of his reading, and by developing flexible theoretical concepts of human development.

SOCIAL AMENITIES

As stated before, a therapeutic session resembles ordinary social interaction in the exchange of words and the observations of all the culturally determined forms of beginning and ending a conversation. The same basic principles of showing respect and courtesy apply. The first step in meeting the stranger who comes to you as a patient, of course, is to introduce yourself and to greet him. However disturbed or reluctant a patient may appear, you should introduce yourself so that you are sure your name has been understood, and you should also ask the patient's name and how he likes to be addressed. I personally have grave misgivings about the habit of addressing an adult patient by first name right from the beginning; this is justified only after a certain degree of intimacy has developed. You should also define your function and state in a few sentences what you know about the patient. If he has been referred by another physician, the name of Dr. X should be mentioned with a brief summary of what he has said or written about the patient and his needs. This step is very important because it gives the patient a chance to correct possible misinformation.

The same applies to children. However suspicious or negatively they may behave, they respond well to being treated with serious courtesy, such as introducing yourself and asking the child's name, telling him what his parents or school or pediatrician have reported about his unhappiness, and explaining how you hope to be of use to him. I recall a six-year-old boy: treatment had been requested by his school because he was extremely shy and withdrawn, practically mute. Rather unexpectedly he entered quite eagerly into play therapy and also made many relevant verbal comments. After some time I asked him what had happened, why he behaved so much more freely here than in school. He answered, "The way you talk; I knew you knew I wasn't dumb."

I received the same explanation from a seventy-eight-year-old woman whom I saw on an emergency basis the day before a Labor Day weekend, at the request of her internist who found her so severely depressed in his office that he felt she might need hospitalization. Not knowing anything about this woman I felt some concern about having to ask so many initial questions. But she answered them appropriately, and with increasing animation. This day was the anniversary of her husband's death, and she expressed guilt for having given permission for an operation of which he had died, at the age of eighty-four. A simple explanation was given, that the responsibility for an operation rested with the surgeon, not with the relative who signs the release. A few other aspects of her background and their possible relationship to her depression were briefly clarified. We decided together that she should go ahead with her plan to spend the weekend in the country, with a companion and some friends, instead of going to a hospital. When I saw her after the weekend the acute depression and anxiety had lessened to a considerable degree. Her explanation was simple: "I felt you thought of me as somebody who could understand complicated things, and not just as a wealthy old lady who wanted attention and needed pampering." She had suffered repeatedly from depressive reactions; when she was in her sixties she had "discovered" psychoanalysis and benefited greatly from working with a therapist who, however, died before her problems were resolved. She had tried to find another therapist but each time was given discouraging explanations that not much could be expected at her age, that psychoanalysis worked best with young people. The experience of my having talked openly about her problems, without any reference to her age, had encouraged her, and she insisted on continuing in therapy, with remarkably positive results.

LIVING CONDITIONS

A common omission of beginners is failure to clarify the conditions under which a patient lives and the circumstances that have led him to seek psychotherapy. I find it useful to explore in some detail what preceded his coming for a consultation, who suggested psychotherapy to him, what treatment he had been exposed to in the past and what it meant to him. I also find it useful to obtain from my office patients, and if possible from hospitalized patients, the kind of information usually taken in part by a secretary, such as address and telephone number, occupation, who is paying the bill, who lives in the household, what kind of neighborhood it is, the style of living, how many bedrooms and what the sleeping arrangements are, how often they have moved, whether relatives live in the home or nearby, whether household help is available, what schools are in the district, and so on. Most patients recognize that this is an "innocent" way of getting acquainted, and it also helps in forming a picture of the patient's social environment and cultural background. All too often beginners get deeply involved in therapy with a patient without having a clear picture of how and where he lives, sometimes not even knowing whether it is difficult and time-consuming for him to come to the office.

There are patients who will react to such a factual inquiry with some annoyance, thinking it a waste of time on trivia or an unnecessary repetition of information already given. Usually such a reaction gives a hint of difficulties ahead. There are people who are determined to talk about big, abstract issues only, who intellectualize about their difficulties but are reluctant to let the true facts about their lives be known or to reveal anything truly personal about themselves. When a patient is disoriented or markedly anxious and depressed, the first task is, of course, to let him talk about his problems and to postpone this type of inquiry to a more propitious time.

FORMAL PROFESSIONAL ARRANGEMENTS

An important part of the initial interview is arranging for the formal aspects of therapy which designate it as a professional relationship, such as determining the frequency of the meetings, the length of each session, and the fee. I find it practical to schedule the first few meetings longer than ordinary sessions, so that there is sufficient time to discuss these practical questions in detail as an important aspect of therapy, not as something that is rushed through in a few minutes at the end. Quite often several sessions will be needed, and it is useful to have them close together, to evaluate the underlying psychological issues along with the relevant practical aspects. One also needs to evaluate a patient's capacity to carry over from one session to another.

Whether treatment can be carried out effectively on a once-a-week basis or whether two or three sessions per week are needed depends not only on the psychological problems but also on a patient's capacity to experience a sense of continuity about being in treatment. There is probably no more revealing expression about the lack of such a sense than inquiries about how many more "treatments" are needed.

The length of the treatment session has traditionally been the "fifty-minute hour" whereby the remaining ten minutes are set aside for the therapist's own use: for reflection on what has gone on, for note taking, and for a breathing spell. This interval also permits a session to run overtime for a few minutes when the material demands it, and to give a patient the chance to recover his equilibrium after an upsetting session without the feeling of being shuttled out because there is another patient waiting to have his allotted minutes. A tendency developed to cut the sessions down to forty-five minutes and to omit the interval altogether. This is effective from an economic angle because then four patients can be seen in a three-hour period. However, this may lead to a rather rushed atmosphere throughout the session and may inhibit a patient in dealing with important and painful material. Such overtight scheduling is particularly damaging to a young therapist because he needs the extra time for reflecting on the session and for evaluating his own behavior and responses.

There is nothing sacred about the fifty- or forty-five-minute hour; it is not the optimal period in all circumstances. The length of a treatment session should be adjusted to a patient's needs. With severe depression, and sometimes with acutely disturbed schizophrenics, shorter and more frequent sessions may be more fruitful. On the other hand, some deeply inhibited patients, borderline schizophrenics, or obsessives may warm up only gradually and may benefit from longer treatment sessions. Much of this can be worked out only as therapy progresses; it is important to keep the need for flexibility in mind. A more experienced and secure therapist will give himself and his patients sufficient time to work in an individualistic way, whereas a beginner may feel obliged to adhere to what he feels is the official and therefore right time.

Whatever schedule has been worked out, once it is made it is important that appointments are kept regularly and on time. Missing appointments or lateness demands an explanation, and the exploration may reveal impractical or unrealistic planning—then a change is indicated. In other patients, being late expresses a reluctance to come or hurt or angry feelings. Sometimes it is a form of self-assertion. But any stereotyped interpretation of lateness would be misleading. I have known very rigid obsessives in whom the first sign that something was maybe loosening up was their being a few minutes late.

The need to be punctual applies just as much to the therapist, if not more so. It is so important that there should be no need to mention it; if nothing else, to be there on time is a matter of courtesy and respect. To keep a patient waiting is not only sloppy carelessness, but also expresses disregard for the importance that the therapeutic session has for a patient who has made an effort to be there on time and who may be anxious about the painful problems he needs to face. Keeping him waiting and to deal with that cavalierly is cruel disregard for a patient's needs and suffering. It is also an indication that a therapist is not taking himself seriously. A beginner may find it hard to believe that the hour really matters to the patient, that he often arranges his whole life around this experience, and that whatever his apparent reluctance and resistance there is a deep-felt need of sharing his suffering with somebody reliable who is truly interested in him. Nothing is more apt to cancel out the experience of a trustworthy and supportive relationship than a therapist who is haphazard in fulfilling his side of the arrangement.

For anxious and depressed people it may be of help to know that the therapist can be reached by telephone; also of help when for practical reasons, such as distance, the number of sessions must be kept to a minimum. Definite instructions should be given when to call and when *not* to. If integrated into the treatment plan, the telephone can play an important role. It is, however, capable of misuse by manipulative patients who, with uncanny perception, will claim an emergency whenever the therapist is resting or is engaged in some important personal activity. A Catholic patient who suffered from tormenting doubts about going, or not going, to confession phoned at 3:00 A.M. on an Easter Sunday, just to tell me that I had been wrong: her refusal to go to confession had nothing to do with her relationship to her mother (who constantly told her she was committing a mortal sin) but reflected a philosophical belief. The simple question, "Why could this information not have waited until your next appointment?" brought home to her that conflicting emotions and bitter feelings were involved.

During an interruption of treatment, as for summer vacation, it is useful to suggest that a patient write down what troubles him, or how he reacts to important events, and to mail these notes to the therapist, not as a formal letter or in the expectation of starting a correspondence, but in order to feel a sense of communication.

THE FEE

Of equal importance to a realistic and reliable time schedule is the setting of a reasonable fee. For hospitalized patients this is usually done on admission through the registrar, though in some hospitals the psychotherapist may make individual fee arrangements with a patient. In private practice fee arrangements are a matter of course, but this aspect is often neglected in out-patient clinics. Student therapists are apt to leave it to the registrar, or they mechanically follow a fee schedule. To arrive at a reasonable and equitable fee actually requires evaluation of a patient's whole style of living, of his attitude toward money and his sense of responsibility. To an amazing degree, difficulties in money matters parallel difficulties in interpersonal relations during the therapy.

The beginner, not thinking very highly of his skills, is apt to set too low a fee, or he fails to pay attention to its being paid regularly. Sometimes there is a marked discrepancy between official and actual income, and a literal interpretation of a fee schedule may distort the whole picture. I recall supervising the treatment of a young woman who was unusually nonserious, even playful, about making use of her treatment time. She was a student teacher and her husband a graduate student, both on very low incomes. Accordingly, she was charged the lowest fee at that time, something like fifty cents a session. Later it was learned that she was the daughter of a very wealthy family; though she and her husband had a separate small apartment, she spent most of her time at her parents' lavish home. On inquiry it was learned that she gave the doorman who called a taxi to take her to the clinic a tip exactly equal to what she paid for her therapeutic session.

In contrast, I recall at about the same time a foreign student, a displaced person who was without resources whatsoever and who supported himself as a hospital technician, without making it clear that this was night work of a few hours only; he was charged five dollars for each session, three times a week. This sum represented about half of his income, and he lived at a poverty level but was too proud to mention it. This was realized only when the therapist noted the complete absence of any recreational activities. There is some old tradition that a fee should be high enough to hurt, to remind the patient of the seriousness of treatment, that it should represent some form of sacrifice. My feeling is that it should be an appropriate sum: not a handout or a charitable token, but not so high either that, as he becomes freer and more capable of enjoying life, a patient is deprived of the means to make use of his newfound freedom.

Beginners frequently fail to notice whether arrangements are adhered to and payments made regularly. Once payment has been omitted, patients are apt to slip into nonpayment over a lengthy period and may accumulate unmanageable debts. There may be legitimate reasons for nonpayment, which will come into the open when the issue is discussed. This may lead to a reconsideration of the fee or to practical planning in view of an unexpected obligation, and such. Regular payment is of importance for a variety of reasons, the most important being that only in this way does the patient feel that the time is truly *his,* to be used in a way that serves his needs, when he can feel free to express whatever feelings come up, including criticism of the therapist or other negative and violent emotions.

Nonattention to payment may conceal serious defects in the progress of therapy. I recall reviewing the treatment performance of a resident who had been in general practice and had decided on a psychiatric career because he had always felt a deep interest in the personal problems of his patients. He was satisfied with his progress as a psychiatrist and showed a warm and protective attitude toward his patients, all of whom came regularly. As it turned out, not one of his patients had paid a single fee in the course of nearly a year, and little of what one might call dynamic therapeutic intervention had taken place with any patient. What had developed was a cozy mutual confidentiality, but without the exploration of any troublesome issues.

A LITERARY EXAMPLE

A detailed description of a first interview can be found in *I Never Promised You a Rose Garden,* a young schizophrenic girl's account of her therapeutic journey. Having been exposed to many previous consultations and treatment efforts, she is extremely suspicious of the new experience, about being hospitalized and being sent for therapy to an elderly woman whom she mistakes at first for the housekeeper. I quote from the book:

They went into a sunny room and the Housekeeper-Famous-Doctor turned, saying, "Sit down. Make yourself comfortable." There came a great exhaustion and when the doctor said, "Is there anything you want to tell me?" a great gust of anger, so that Deborah stood up quickly . . . "All right—you'll ask me questions and I'll answer them—you'll clear up my 'symptoms' and then send me home . . . *and what will I have then?*"

The doctor said quietly, "If you did not really want to give them up, you wouldn't tell me . . . Come, sit down. You will not have to give up anything until you are ready, and then there will be something to take its place . . . Do you know why you are here?"*

There follows an outburst of a long list of self-belittling descriptions, with expressed anger that her complaints had been rated imaginary. The patient feels that she has spoken her true feelings for the first time.

The doctor said simply, "Well, that seems to be quite a list. Some of these things, I think, are not so, but we have a job cut out for us."

"To make me friendly and sweet and agreeable and happy in the lies I tell."

"To help you to get well."

"To shut up the complaints."

"To end them, where they are the products of an upheaval in your feelings."

The rope tightened. Fear was flowing wildly in Deborah's head, turning her vision gray. "You're saying what they all say—phony complaints about nonexistent sicknesses."

* Hannah Green, *I Never Promised You a Rose Garden* (New York: Holt, Rinehart and Winston, 1964), pp. 24–25.

"It seems to me that I said you are very sick, indeed."

"Like the rest of them here?" . . .

"Do you mean to ask me if I think you belong here, if yours is what is called a mental illness? Then the answer is yes. I think you are sick in this way, but with your very hard work here and with a doctor's working hard with you, I think you can get better." (pp. 25–26)

I am sure I do not divulge a professional secret when I mention that Dr. Fried, the therapist in the story, was Dr. Frieda Fromm-Reichmann. Never having treated an adolescent, she asked me to stand by as a consultant and to meet her young patient. Years later, as treatment approached successful termination, Fromm-Reichmann, as was her custom, reviewed with her patient what she herself had considered most helpful and significant for the recovery. I report it here as I heard it from Fromm-Reichmann. When questioned the girl said, "You shouldn't ask, doctor. It was the WE experience . . . don't you remember, doctor, the first day, when I said, you will take away my gut pain, you will take away my trances and you will take away my food, and *what will I have then?* . . . Don't you remember what you said . . . you did *not* say 'I will not take it away' . . . You said, 'You come and tell me about all of this—that tells me that you do not want it. What I hear is that you want *us* to free you from them.' I tell you, doctor, that word *us* did the trick. Here was somebody who did not think she could cure me, or do it for me, but who said, 'We'll do it together.' "

There are other aspects of the initial interview which this patient experiences as encouraging, namely the doctor's honest answer when asked about the seriousness of the illness. This gives her a feeling of relief; it was the end of all the "there is nothing the matter with you" rounds of doctors. Here at last was a vindication of all her anger in all those offices. In the patient's own account the therapist notes this relaxation, asks about it, and receives a schizophrenic answer:

"I am thinking about the difference between a misdemeanor and a felony."

"How so?"

"The prisoner pleads guilty to the charge of not having acute something-itis and accepts the verdict of guilty of being nuts in the first degree."

"Perhaps in the second degree," the doctor said, smiling a little. "Not entirely voluntarily nor entirely with forethought." (p. 26)

Beginners are often worried about not knowing enough, about not being able to explain things immediately. This account of a first interview describes clearly the essential task: to listen with an honest and open mind, to convey to a patient that one is available for his journey of self-discovery but with the implication, from the very beginning, that this can be successful only when both take part in the work of this journey together.

2

Personality in the Making

As a guide for how to proceed and what to look for, where and when to intervene, the therapist needs some theoretical orientation to help him evaluate the factors that have contributed to his patient's difficulties. Psychotherapy rests on the assumption that problems with an origin in damaging and confusing early experiences are capable of correction through a new and different intimate personal relationship.

There has been an unending and continuous debate whether mental illness is caused by genetic or other organic factors or should be attributed to psychological stress. Traditionally the problem was posed as an either/or question, with the implication that genetic endowment and life experience were mutually exclusive. Modern biological research has taught us that the characteristics of each particular person have a basis in his genetic endowment; however, human personality does not evolve merely from the unfolding of these innate traits, and early experiences are essential for the organization and differentiation of these potentialities. Even now there are some who do not recognize the interaction of the organic and psychological aspects, and who continue to contrast an organic cause of psychiatric illness with a psychodynamic origin. Those who tend to attribute everything to hereditary factors rarely are interested in a psychotherapeutic approach; nor are they effective when they attempt it, even after admitting that major environmental factors may have played a role in the development of a particular illness.

Those with a definite interest in the psychological aspects of mental illness, and who conceive of personality as having evolved from the interaction of biological givens with ongoing life experiences, also encounter difficulties. They may find it confusing that they have to choose between competing theoretical constructs in order to find one suited to their particular style of thinking. A student therapist may feel himself the victim of endless and seemingly unsoluble controversies when he seeks to organize his observations and experiences. Psychotherapeutic principles and insights are most effectively learned firsthand, and no amount of instruction and reading can replace the vitality of learning by doing. Each therapist must experience as real a patient's struggles to bring into the open topics that are difficult or painful to face, and he must learn to recognize his own reactions during this process. At the same time, he must perform an intellectual task, that of recognizing more generalized principles that may be deduced from what he observes in individual sessions and that will be helpful in broadening the range of his perception.

It is a puzzling fact that in this search for theoretical principles the student, in many training programs, is not offered up-to-date information on child development and personality growth, and on how disturbances in this process may result in emotional and mental difficulties. Instead he is frankly indoctrinated with a preferred theory as expressed by different "schools" of psychiatry. Most often he is taught elaborate but outdated psychoanalytic principles. As a result, he is forever worried about the relevance of his own observations, whether or not they fit a particular theory, and cannot approach each patient with an uncluttered mind, motivated only by the desire to learn.

Dynamic psychotherapy is a direct descendant of psychoanalysis, and some of its basic tenets are identical with what is taught and practiced as psychoanalysis. Since they were first formulated, psychoanalytic principles have undergone many changes and elaborations, and the whole field has come under increasing scrutiny. Much of what Freud taught has stood the test of time. Probably his greatest contribution is his recognition that abnormal mental phenomena carry various symbolic meanings and can be understood. He did this at a time when being scientific as a psychiatrist was conceived of only in one way—as looking for some definite organic cause. It was a revolutionary step when he focused psychiatric interest on the individual person with mental problems, and when he developed a therapeutic method on the basis of this understanding. There is also general agreement with his formulation of the "genetic principle," that the degree of mental health or ill health is closely related to intimate aspects of early life experiences. We also owe to Freud our awareness of "transference phenomena," that the doctor-patient relationship involves many irrational aspects, unexamined carry-overs from childhood experiences and attachments, and that their clarification is an important step in resolving conflicts. Specifically Freud's name is associated with our knowledge that the most troublesome sources of psychic disequilibrium are "unconscious," outside of awareness, and that these hidden elements need to be made conscious so that they can be reexamined and thus brought into line with rational adult thinking.

PSYCHOANALYTIC THEORY

These basic principles, however, are not generally taught in simple everyday language and in a way that the student can bring his observations into harmony with them; they are enmeshed in a bewildering maze of all the variations that psychoanalytic theory has undergone since its first formulation seventy or eighty years ago. It is nearly axiomatic to say that in order to do psychotherapy one must have a solid knowledge of "psychodynamics," that is, explanations based on psychoanalytic theory. And this is where some of the difficulties begin. In order to keep matters simple, these elaborate theoretical abstractions are not offered as what they are, as provisional attempts to deal with complex issues which are often difficult to define and are expressed in the picturesque language of analogies; they are presented as "basic scientific facts," with an embarrassing tendency to compare "the psychodynamics" with the laws of physics, as if that would make them "scientific." Many concepts and terms have become part of the everyday thinking and speech of educated people, and they have acquired the traditional odor of venerability—but that does not make them facts.

Psychoanalysis and its theoretical formulations have undergone enormous changes during the last few decades. There has been an endless stream of publications dealing with "advances," "progress," or "modification" in psychoanalytic technique. Few papers state openly that such changes indicate that the earlier concepts were associated with unsatisfactory treatment results. Not uncommonly, Freud's earliest concepts and deductions are offered as established facts, and the beginner may proceed along the lines of a classical psychoanalytic model that has long been abandoned by experienced workers in the field.

The concept of "psychodynamics" has been endowed with a quasi-magical significance, and its components are often memorized in the hope of gaining a better understanding of different clinical pictures or symptom complexes. In his efforts to identify "the psychodynamics" or "defense mechanisms," the therapist may only see psychological bits and pieces and fail to approach his patient with an open mind and sympathy for the suffering of the particular individual. The discrepancy between the commonly taught theoretical elaborations and the beginner's factual experiences makes "learning psychotherapy" seem a bewildering, even impossible, task.

I shall present here the assumptions underlying classic psychoanalytic theory in a deliberately oversimplified form. In its structure and imagery the theory conceives of the infant as born equipped with instincts that if allowed to flourish, not deformed through the vicissitudes of the repressive culture, would guide an individual to a healthy, nonneurotic life. Specifically the sexual instinct, the libido, suffers from these damaging cultural prohibitions, and thus becomes fixated at various levels of psychosexual development. The instinctual repression results in unconscious conflicts which become manifest as neurotic symptoms. Psychoanalytic therapy, in this classical model, consists of uncovering the repressed conflicts, invariably of a sexual nature, and the psychic trauma that caused them. Making such conflicts conscious, by working through transference and resistance, was expected to bring about a cure through liberation of the libido and through insight into the repressed memories. Freud presented these fundamental concepts as an elaborate theory of instincts, also called libido theory, in the language of metaphors. Throughout his life he struggled to revise the theory, and he remained critical of all his efforts to formulate a fixed theory of instincts; yet many of his early followers accepted his theoretical assumptions as proven facts—and passed them on as such to subsequent generations.

Psychoanalytic thinking has changed considerably, away from the model of the organism as a closed system inhabited by powerful instincts to much more operational concepts—namely of the individual in functional interaction with people in his environment. As the theoretical concepts changed, the technique of treatment moved away from the model of the therapist as a blank mirror reflecting a patient's free associations to which he would give meaning through his interpretations. In modern psychoanalytic thinking, therapy is conceived of as a significant interaction between patient and therapist which ultimately leads to corrective changes in the patient's personality; this definition is identical with what is practiced as dynamic psychotherapy. The great puzzle is the longevity and survival of the outmoded model, which has led too many a beginner to approach a patient with the passive "say-everything-that-comes-to-your-mind" attitude, without acknowledging what he hears a patient say or guiding him to greater clarity through appropriate questions.

MISUSE OF TERMINOLOGY

This confusing traditionalism can be explained, in part at least, by the fact that, with all the changes in basic concepts, the vocabulary invented to convey the meaning of the earliest psychoanalytic formulations continues to be used. Each new generation of students has to struggle to get at the underlying meaning, or he will defend his new knowledge as a sacred possession. There are many who would feel diminished in their professional standing if they were to refer to "infancy" just like that, instead of calling it the "oral phase," or to difficulties in early life by an exact description of what they have reconstructed, instead of referring to them as "problems in orality." One could cite endless examples where professional clichés are used instead of the ordinary word. Many would feel it beneath their dignity to refer to a child during the school years other than as a "latency child." I have asked many students why they referred to people as "objects": they were not aware that this term was a fossil from the earliest days of psychoanalysis, when interaction between people was seen as the libido searching to attach itself to "an object." Many other terms that originally had a rather definite meaning continue to be in use even though the underlying concepts have changed. Experienced analysts are quite aware of the changes in meaning, although I have still to find any two who would agree about the exact meaning and significance of the changes.

Not uncommonly a beginner will become a "true believer" to resolve his doubts and uncertainties. He will be reluctant to follow a theoretical model that is less prestigious even though it might be more helpful for him in organizing his work. The traditional teaching of psychoanalytic principles, or the way a beginner understands them, may result in his becoming preoccupied with "theory," and this can stand in the way of open-minded observations. Young psychiatrists are apt to acquire an extensive psychoanalytic vocabulary, and this excess verbiage may act like shining but distorting glasses: the beginner can misperceive what is going on with a patient and will classify him according to some preconceived notion about "psychodynamics." Instead of sympathetically observing and responding to his patient's behavior and utterances, he will label him with accusing, punitive, and essentially invalidating epitaphs—"passive-aggressive," "masochistic," "compulsive," "latent homosexual," and so on. The less secure a therapist is, the more likely he will cling to stereotyped concepts and a cliché-ridden vocabulary. In some the quest for certainty and definite rules persists through the training period, with a rigid adherence to old psychoanalytic concepts as "basic facts." Sooner or later a student must come to terms with the plain unalterable fact that there are no definite complexes or psychodynamics to be recognized in all his cases, no definite rules which, if rigidly applied, will turn him into an effective therapist.

Some of my colleagues feel that my concern with the excessive use of psychiatric clichés is unjustified, that modern teachers avoid throwing such stereotyped concepts at students. It still does occur, though, and I should like to cite a recent episode. In a seminar on psychotherapy a medical student complained to the class that he had not understood what his supervisor meant when he told him what the matter was with his patient and what he should say to her; he added that he had been annoyed at being instructed in such an authoritarian way. His patient was a twenty-two-year-old woman who was depressed because her third marriage was breaking up. She had quite a long list of complaints about the inadequacies of her various husbands. Her own parents had been divorced when she was five years old, and she had always blamed her mother for this, not the father. She knew something was wrong about her reaction because she had been told that her father had been involved with another woman and that this was the reason for the divorce. When the student discussed this with the instructor, he was told that it was an unresolved Oedipus complex and he should confront his patient with it. Several students commented that this was the type of thing that turned them off psychiatry; it made no sense to them. They were familiar with the common definition of the Oedipus complex, that a little boy wants to marry his mother and kill his father, but they were skeptical about looking for this constellation in every case, even in girls.

I agreed with the students that such a highly complex and controversial term was of little help in teaching one how to proceed, but said that dissatisfaction with a term does not mean that there are no important psychological issues needing clarification—they can be elucidated if the therapist has a clear concept of what to look for. Every small child develops an intense emotional attachment to his parents, regardless of the objective qualities of their character and behavior. Not uncommonly a father and his little daughter take particular delight in each other, and his leaving would be a painful loss for her. At age five a child still experiences the world in unrealistic terms, and this little girl had probably retained an exaggerated concept of a father's role, that he could and would do everything for her. In view of his complete absence later on, and with the probability that the mother had not been very helpful and supportive, this girl never had the opportunity to reevaluate her childish expectations of what a man should do for her. The students took an active part in formulating questions that might clarify this situation, so that the young woman could be brought to an understanding of how this childhood loss had left her with unrealistic expectations. The students felt that this unmystical, down-to-earth discussion had helped them grasp what psychotherapy was about, or at least one aspect of it.

Subsequently I discussed this incident with a group of first-year psychiatric residents, who agreed that it was poor teaching to give this concept to a medical student because "he would not know what it means." But when asked what the term meant to them, not one was able to give a definition that had relevance to the data at hand, except that an emotional trauma when a child was five years old implies that it was "Oedipal." They obviously felt that it was more professional for them as psychiatrists to express themselves in established phrases and to approach the particular from the general, however poorly they understood the generalization.

THE INTERPERSONAL THEORY OF PSYCHIATRY

Disagreeing with established theory has never been treated generously in psychoanalysis, regardless of numerous efforts to revise and broaden certain concepts. The censorship is equally repressive today when we are dealing with such far-reaching changes that Freud himself would probably not recognize them as expressing his Theory. Only acknowledged authorities are permitted to express new ideas, and observations and contributions by others are strictly ignored until the signal is finally given to integrate such new knowledge into the theory. In the 1930s many European psychoanalysts openly began to express their concern with the inadequacies of existing theory. These innovations stayed essentially within the conceptual framework and terminology of the original theory. They made their way to

America only slowly, and integration into psychiatric teaching took even longer. The fact that the vocabulary used to express the assumptions of the original theory was retained demanded rather involved reasoning and verbal manipulation to incorporate the new ideas while expressing reverence for the old and established.

Much more sweeping were the revisions formulated during the 1930s and 1940s by Harry Stack Sullivan, one of the early American psychoanalysts, whose psychotherapeutic work with schizophrenics had convinced him that some of the early assumptions were untenable. He subsequently discarded the whole psychoanalytic terminology as misleading neologisms based on unprovable assumptions which, he felt, might interfere with effective therapy. His essential innovation does not rest in his agreeing or disagreeing with one or another aspect of theory, but in his knowingly using a conceptual framework derived from developments in modern physics. The orthodox psychoanalytic theory is formulated by the deterministic conceptual thinking of old-time physics. In the new orientation, phenomena are no longer explained as occurring in an isolated closed organism and according to deterministic, one cause/one effect concepts. Sullivan stressed that the changes in scientific thinking, which at that time were formulated as field theory, needed to be applied to psychiatry. Accordingly, human behavior should no longer be explained in terms of isolated events but as processes resulting from the interaction of multiple forces within a prevailing field. Such changes in conceptual thinking require redefinition in operational terms of the whole field of psychiatric study, of child development, and of the psychotherapeutic process.

Sullivan's ideas have been incorporated into American psychiatric thinking to such an extent that some may ask, "What is so special about Sullivan? These are things we all do and know about." Much of what is published even now as original and new, as radical departure from the traditional psychoanalytic "intrapsychic" model, can be traced to him. Whether we speak of milieu therapy or the whole field of social psychiatry, or whether we are engaged in detailed family studies or express modern psychoanalytic thinking as "object-relationship theory," or whether we are interested in linguistics and the significance of communication, the roots of these and many other developments in psychiatry can readily be recognized in Sullivan's teaching.

Sullivan conceived of "personality" not as a static or stable entity but as an abstraction, as referring to the "relatively enduring patterns of recurrent interpersonal situations which characterize the human life." The organization and integration of such patterns begin at the moment of birth and signify the transformation of the newborn, the purely physiological human organism that Sullivan called "man the animal," into a person. Though dependent on and limited by inborn biological factors, the significant differences in human personality are predominantly determined by individual interpersonal experiences. No one biological drive, sexual or otherwise, could possibly be thought of as the sole cause of the endless variations of human motivation and behavior. Instead he focused on the actions and feeling states of the people who are in continuous interaction with the developing infant.

Sullivan organized his observations and theoretical deductions around the concept of *experience,* the *inner* component of any event and of anything that is lived and is not identical with the *outer* event in which the organism participates. This integration of experiences occurs in *different modes* of conceptualization, depending on the state of maturity of the individual and also on the quality of his interpersonal relatedness. A large part of therapy is taken up with recognizing and correcting the expressions of immature "parataxic" experiences which interfere with realistic appraisals of events and of oneself in relation to others.

Sullivan differentiated tension states in the physical-chemical organism as need for *satisfaction,* and the tension of anxiety as need for interpersonal *security.* He conceived of the infant as born with almost full physiological functions, including the capacity for emotional reactions, but as helplessly dependent on others for the satisfaction of his bodily needs. He stressed that at no time could an infant be considered apart from the setting in which he lived. Optimal development requires that the attainment of satisfaction is association with approval from the significant person, which is experienced as a sense of well-being or security. If there is no appropriate response to his needs, if there is strain, frustration, or disapproval, his state of well-being will be disturbed; this is experienced as *anxiety,* a profound feeling of uneasiness and discomfort. This experience of anxiety, or the need to avoid it, is the dynamic force that molds each individual into a definite personality. Only those expressions of his actions, motivations, thoughts, and desires that meet with approval from the significant people, and thus do not provoke the disintegrating experience of anxiety, develop within his range of awareness, and become capable of mature, rational usage. Sullivan called this part of the personality, experienced as "I" or "myself," the self-system, and its function is to screen the permissible and approved from the forbidden and disapproved. If the child is exposed to severe disapproval, the self-dynamism will develop into a harsh and rigid instrument, hemmed in by anxiety at every step, excluding from awareness the corrective and broadening experiences that are essential for healthy personality growth. Such a person will suffer from low self-esteem and will have a great capacity for finding fault with himself and others; to the extent that he misinterprets reality, he must be considered mentally ill.

Though Sullivan elaborated the significance and vicissitudes of interpersonal experiences during infancy and early childhood in great detail, he emphasized also the importance of the juvenile and preadolescent period for corrective experiences. If not too severely handicapped, a child will be able to find help in emerging from family bonds and in developing a more realistic and competent self-concept, through the experience of intimacy in a meaningful friendship.

Sullivan redefined the role of the therapist as that of a participant-observer, in contrast to the blank-mirror image of the classical psychoanalyst. He viewed the therapeutic situation as a particular kind of interpersonal relationship with a definite purpose, that of ensuring increased skills of living for the patient. The special skill of the psychiatrist is his alert attention to phenomena that distort the ongoing life processes. In his teaching Sullivan emphasized how to clarify underlying disturbances, how and where to look, but without outlining what one would find—that he expected to differ from one individual to another. Minor manifestations of anxiety serve as a guide and stimulus for relevant inquiry in uncovering dissociated aspects of current and past distorting experiences. He warned against prematurely confronting a patient with what the therapist has assumed to be the problem, because of the danger of precipitating severe anxiety. Annoying, irritating, or hostile expressions need to be respected as signals of severe underlying anxiety or a conviction of inner worthlessness. Sullivan described the basic therapeutic attitude as the need to consider a patient, regardless of how seriously disturbed he might appear, "more human than otherwise."

MODERN STUDIES OF EARLY DEVELOPMENT

The first theories of personality were reconstructed from patients' accounts of their childhood experiences. Modern concepts are increasingly based on direct observations of infants: how they grow into mature, though to some extent disturbed, individuals and how this occurs in interaction with the mother and other significant people in the family and in the wider social and cultural setting. Some early direct observations were still restricted by their use to confirm psychoanalytic constructs. Such efforts have been abandoned, and some significant reformulations have come from formerly "classical" psychoanalysts.

An important expression of the concern with objectivity is the incorporation of Jean Piaget's work into dynamic psychiatric thinking. Early analysts rejected his work as too conceptual, unconcerned with emotional experiences. Sullivan had anticipated in his concept of increasingly maturing "modes of experience" what Piaget subsequently documented in great detail. It is now generally acknowledged that observations on thinking and behavior during childhood cannot be understood without an intimate knowledge of the changes in mental capacity of infants and children. According to Piaget, these changing conceptual stages are integrated in a dual way: one he calls "accommodation," the transformation induced in the child's perceptual schemata and behavior patterns by the environment; the other is "assimilation," the incorporation of objects and characteristics of the environment into the child's patterns of perception and behavior. Piaget conceives of the child as actively working on the integration of new mental structures. In early psychoanalytic thinking "pleasure" was viewed as the gratification of instinctual drives; Piaget defines it in active terms as "being the cause of something."

I am in the habit of asking residents what they have considered useful in the teaching process. Recently one answered, without hesitation, "psychoanalytic theory." When asked what specifically had been helpful he gave as example, "what Piaget had said about learning by doing and repeating" and the way this was expressed in the conceptual thinking of children. He was rather surprised when told that Piaget probably would be pleased that his teaching had been useful to a young psychiatrist, but that he certainly would not be flattered to be grouped with psychoanalysts.

Modern studies and direct observations have shown that a wide range of other functions and faculties in the newborn infant are much less organized than had been assumed, and that for proper integration there is need for confirming and reinforcing responses from the mother and others in the environment; without this, deficits in various functional activities will result. Extreme deficits in patterns of adaptation and behavior have been observed in infant monkeys who were removed from their mothers at birth and were raised in complete isolation. At about one year they were placed together with other monkeys of the same age, which did not help to correct the early deficits. When fully grown they were grossly abnormal, apathetic, stereotyped in their responses, inadequate in sexual behavior though they had undergone normal physiological puberty. They also exhibited many bizarre mouthing habits and were deficient in their ability to regulate their food intake.

In human development deprivation is rarely this extreme, but many observations indicate that inappropriate responses in the parent-child interaction result in deficiencies not only in psychological reactions but also in the organization of bodily functions and the awareness of somatic sensations. In the older models, the infant was conceived of as fairly well organized biologically but utterly helpless in fulfilling his needs, a passive receiver of adult administrations. These traditional assumptions neglect the fact that the infant, though immature, is also an active participant in his survival; he gives clues and signals indicating states of discomfort and unfulfilled needs. How they are responded to, whether gratified or disregarded, appears to be the critical influence on his becoming conscious of what his needs are. The human infant starts life with biological urges that, in his subjective experience, are no more than unidentified and unidentifiable states of tension and discomfort, and he is unable to differentiate himself from others. The sense of separateness evolves from interactional processes that in a crucial way foreshadow his later sense of effective identity. Healthy or distorted development is shaped, to a large extent, by the appropriateness of a mother's response to expressions of needs, in the psychological as well as the biological area. If confirmation and reinforcement of his own initially rather undifferentiated sensations are absent, or contradictory or inaccurate, then a child will grow up without the essential groundwork for developing "body identity," without perceptual and conceptual awareness of his own abilities and functions, particularly when he tries to differentiate between biological and emotional disturbances. He will be apt to misinterpret deformities in his self-body concept as externally induced. The most severe form of such maldevelopment occurs in schizophrenics who fail to identify or respond to their needs and feel helpless under the influence of external forces.

Various studies have focused on disturbances in what has been called the "circular and reciprocal feedback patterns of interaction," and have focused on different areas of maldevelopment in different phases of childhood. Traditionally the development of autonomy and individuation has been attributed to late infancy and the toddler stage. In my experience these patterns begin to establish themselves practically at the moment of birth and can be observed directly in the feeding situation. Inappropriate feeding, with a mother superimposing her concepts of what the child needs instead of taking the cues from him, is associated with severe deficits in initiative and self-directiveness. Later maldevelopment has to do with a parent's responses to a child's growing independence. Disturbances may result from the compulsion of an immature or insecure parent to mold a child in a way that supplements the parent's own deficiencies, or fulfills his image of being "right." Every mother is concerned about dangers to her child and must teach him how to handle threatening events from the outside; an obsessive mother might attempt to make her child perfect. Many of the older formulations focused on the child's need for sufficient freedom from inhibition and oppression. It is more clearly recognized now that for healthy maturation the development of his inner independence and competence must be encouraged, but also that the demands placed on a child should not precede the degree of his maturation.

Another area that is more clearly recognized today is the influence of correct and meaningful interaction on the development of language and clear conceptual thinking. A continuously inappropriate style of communication on the part of a parent will deprive a child of the help he needs to categorize his various experiences and to interpret correctly other people's responses. Extensive research into the family background of schizophrenics has revealed how deficiencies in the proper use of language are preparation for potential schizophrenic responses. In the long run it matters whether a child gets help from other sources in widening his range of experiences, which then acts to correct early misinterpretations. If his life is too restricted, he will remain confused and erroneous in interpreting other people's behavior, and also in his own self-evaluation. Disturbances in communication play some role in all mental disorders.

According to these concepts, effective therapy must offer a patient assistance in "self-orientation." Therapy must assist in the development of clearer perceptions of what is going on, and in evoking enough awareness of impulses, thoughts, and feelings to allow the insecure person to meet life's problems with less anxiety and greater self-assurance.

THEORY AND THERAPY

I have attempted to present here some theoretical principles of early personality development in a form that will make sense to a beginner, without sidetracking him into the fine points of theoretical controversies. I have found this theoretical frame flexible enough to accommodate a wide range of observations, and it has been useful in helping student therapists to make sensitive and relevant observations with an appreciation for many kinds of appropriate and individualistic responses. If the teaching he gets is dogmatic, then the beginner is in danger of becoming too rigid and narrow in his approach. Submission to unqualified statements may result in a narrowing of vision, whereas an open-minded use of theoretical possibilities will serve to expand horizons. The young therapist may try a literal application of oversimplified dynamics as he understands them, fitting his own observations into a definite theoretical structure, or he may become "eclectic," trying to find the solution in a different theoretical model. When disappointed with treatment results, he may become convinced that theory does not matter, that all depends on his personal qualities, his warmth and friendliness; or, worst of all, he may develop therapeutic nihilism.

During my own residency I had an impressive experience of seeing dramatic improvement in a seemingly untreatable patient, after a change in therapeutic approach based on changed theoretical considerations. Zelda was a woman of twenty-six who had been sick with numerous crippling obsessions, including compulsive hand washing, for over five years; she had been hospitalized for the last two. She appeared preoccupied with the sinfulness of sex and her own hostility, and lived in constant dread of harming others by passing on "germs" to them. These problems had been reviewed with her previous therapists, who seemed to have encouraged her talking along this line.

When she became my patient I presented her history in a seminar to Harry Stack Sullivan, who in his discussion focused on the obsessive's use of verbal maneuvers to keep from dealing with the real underlying problems. Sullivan suggested a change of focus, away from the increasingly fruitless ruminations to an awareness of what was going on in her daily life; all discussion should concentrate on how she felt about the people around her, what experiences she had with them and with her family. Zelda found it difficult to talk about such small events; she expressed concern that we were not dealing with the deeper problems. However, she began to pay attention to the people around her and would talk about them as individuals. She also began to become aware of her own feelings; until then she had spoken of disliking a great many people, was critical of all of them, and was vaguely irritable with no apparent motivation. For a while she was quite confused about her own emotional reactions, often unable to differentiate between like and dislike, love and hate, irritation and friendly interest. The diffuse feelings of hatred for everyone gradually became more differentiated, with awareness of justified anger for specific events or mishaps.

Within a month she appeared more outgoing, became friendly with several other patients, and stopped talking about her germs and the other symptoms that had so preoccupied her. As her overt symptoms diminished, Zelda was able to review her whole development in much more realistic language. She had been continuously worried about what other people thought of her, had always been conscientious about doing everything to perfection; but she had never felt good about anything or able to feel satisfied that it was all right. Now instead of talking in general terms about sex and her hostility, she became increasingly detailed and realistic, with criticism of specific events in reviewing her development and her interaction in the family. The scope of her activities increased greatly and rather rapidly; she began to work in the administrative office, where she proved herself a very competent secretary, and took a more active part in various social and athletic activities. She was able to leave the hospital four months after the change in treatment approach, and she returned to her home after one more month as an out-patient. She kept in touch with me for some time to let me know that the improvement had lasted.

If one wants to account for this dramatic change, several points need to be considered. On first glance we might conclude that it was the change of focus from the past to the here and now. Though this is what was done, it expresses only an incidental aspect of what happened. While examining the events in her current life, Zelda became aware of what she herself felt and experienced; she stopped speculating about assumed feelings of hostility or sexual conflicts and how they related to so-called traumatic events of the past. In the process she became more discriminatingly aware of her own psychological abilities, and she reexamined her childhood experiences with these new tools. She also discovered that she had inner resources and the courage to lead a less guilt-ridden, more self-assertive life.

As a supervisor I have observed over and over again that therapists who focus on their patients' daily lives, and on how they feel about and get along with people, have better treatment results than those who are preoccupied with translating whatever a patient expresses into some kind of professional jargon, or those who conceive of what a patient does or says as productions of the unconscious mind to which he, the therapist, is supposed to give meaning. For uncovering and correcting underlying causes, it is more helpful to begin with the immediate relevant aspects of a patient's malfunctioning, and this should be followed by a gradual reconstruction of the distorting background experiences. To bring about meaningful change, the therapist needs to have clear concepts of the fundamental aspects of the development of psychiatric disorders, but he must always be aware that the specific area and content of an individual's maldevelopment will vary widely from person to person.

3

The World Around

People who undergo psychotherapy do not live in a vacuum. Some may live alone and need help in breaking out of the cage of their isolation. Others live in their parents' home where they may feel hemmed in and controlled; or they may live with their spouse and children, or with a friend or lover, where personal conflicts arise. Those who are more severely disturbed may be hospitalized or live in some sheltered environment, where arrangements are made for them. Not all complaints and difficulties should be attributed to the patient's neuroticism and misinterpretations. A realistic evaluation will often reveal problems that can and should be corrected. Many adhere, though to different degrees, to old prejudices against psychiatry; the very fact that a person is in psychiatric treatment is resented as something embarrassing or shameful. Such attitudes need to be clarified early on, before they become intermingled with problems that invariably arise in the family interaction when a member undergoes psychotherapy.

In the traditional psychoanalytic approach, contact with the family was avoided. If other members appeared to be in need of help, they were referred to another therapist. Such a rigid separation of the patient and members of his family rests on the assumption that each person has his own intrapsychic problems that need to be resolved. Modern theories of personality no longer conceive of the intrapsychic process as something unrelated to the on-going interaction with others, though focus on the patient himself continues to be the preferred approach in individual psychotherapy with adults who seek help on their own for various neurotic problems and difficulties, but who are otherwise in control of their lives. Coming to an understanding of the underlying distorted reactions leads to greater competence in handling these various problems, including those in relation to others. However, not paying attention to the turmoil that mental illness and its treatment evoke for the whole family, even when the patient no longer lives in the same household, frequently accounts for harmful interference by parents or marriage partners. This is more likely to occur when the attitudes of the other family members have not been acknowledged or have been brushed aside.

CONTACT WITH RELATIVES AND ASSOCIATES

Even when the focus is on the patient who comes for treatment, the question of seeing another member of the family may come up. When abnormal behavior continues though the underlying factors seem to have been clarified, one needs to ask what or who keeps it going. Domineering, overcontrolling behavior may be sustained by the submissive or indecisive attitudes of a partner. Sometimes it is the whole family structure that requires one member to be in the sick role.

Whenever contact with others appears indicated, the patient himself should be informed and should be asked for consent. Not uncommonly, concerned relatives will approach the therapist to imply that they have important secret information. This is a situation fraught with danger, and it should be discouraged. Seeing a family member without the knowledge of a patient or, even rarer, against his expressed wishes should be allowed only under exceptional circumstances. The patient, when agreeing to such a conference, should have the privilege of outlining which problems can be taken up with a relative and of deciding what he considers definite "privileged communication" not to be divulged to others. His wishes about what he feels can be shared or not shared should be respected. If a patient lists too many and trivial items as private, this may be an expression of an oversuspicious attitude and the distrust needs to be explored in therapy as a major issue. And the family needs to be informed that, in view of the therapeutic needs of the patient, whatever comes up will be used in later therapeutic sessions, so that the patient can examine with the therapist how he experienced the events the relatives brought up and how he feels they affected him.

The same rule of exercising great care not to reveal anything private about a patient, even the fact that he is a patient, applies to contact with other associates, be they partners in an intimate affair, teachers, coworkers, or employers. Many people in treatment are actively engaged in productive work and keeping therapy a secret may become an issue. Some will go to great lengths and inconvenience to keep the fact that they are in therapy from all supposedly prejudiced people. I remember a young woman who came for treatment because she suffered from recurrent depressions and could not decide whether to pursue a career or to get married. She was a late-born child and lived in the same household with her aged mother, who was a well-known social leader. Both women were socially active and had many and varied obligations. It took major effort and much deceptive planning to hide the regular treatment sessions from the mother. Once, during a bitter argument, the daughter threw it into her mother's face that she was seeing a psychiatrist. Unexpectedly, the old woman exclaimed: "Glory, hallelujah! That's what I felt you needed, only I didn't know how to tell you."

Not uncommonly, work inhibition or complete inability to hold on to a job may be the very reason for treatment. Others may be troubled by uncertainties in deciding on a career; conversely, apathy or indifference, "doing nothing," may be the leading complaint. Questions and situations come up where the therapist may be the one best able to help in making a decision, or the one who has the authority to motivate parents, teachers, or other significant people in helping the patient to take steps toward a more independent life, without increasing the underlying resentments and misunderstandings.

It has been an old tradition to discourage a patient from making decisions on vital issues, such as getting married or divorced or making major career changes, before the underlying neurotic distortions have been clarified. One must be confident that it is a rational decision, not escape from old entanglements or flight into a new version of old ones. This is a rule that has stood the test of time, but today's young patients are reluctant to adhere to it. Whatever the conditions and circumstances under which a patient spends most of his day, there are usually innumerable questions that come up in connection with these practical aspects of living, where the therapist may either feel called upon to take an active stand or refuse to do so. Beginners may be troubled by the question whether such direct participation in the realities of a patient's life is compatible with the psychotherapeutic process. They may be clinging to the old ivory-tower concept of psychoanalysis, whereby therapy is solely the investigation of unconscious processes and transference phenomena, and the idea of being of help in real-life situations is considered "unanalytic."

THERAPEUTIC INVOLVEMENT OF THE FAMILY

There has been increasing recognition that emotional difficulties are as much the outcome of what goes on between people as they are of intrapsychic processes, and correction of the often glaring and damaging environmental influences is an essential aspect of therapy. Though this is particularly apparent when dealing with children and young people or severely disturbed hospitalized patients, all of whom are powerless to make decisions about their lives, contact with the parents or mate may be necessary for clarifying the recurrent entanglements even with people who appear less helpless.

Whether such direct participation in the realities of a patient's life is compatible with the psychotherapeutic process depends on many individualistic circumstances. The therapist must be sure of his ability to assess the situation objectively, according to the patient's and the family's needs, not according to his own preferences. He must also be sure that he does not use such decision making to enhance his own prestige. "Playing God" in other people's lives contradicts the essential therapeutic task.

Marked changes have taken place in the way work with the family is integrated with the psychotherapeutic process, though there are still many unsolved problems. In contrast to avoidance of all contact with relatives, the trend is now toward treating the family as a unit, in conjoint sessions. The reports are full of optimism and enthusiasm, with nearly miraculous transformations of life-long patterns of interaction. Such positive results may be achieved by experienced family therapists who responsibly stand by during the upheavals and crises that are being stirred up, and who also recognize the danger signals when too much hurtful material is exposed too fast. The danger of such conferences with the whole family is that, when the therapist succeeds in making some dramatic point, the participants may feel that they have been tricked into revealing various pathological and guilt-ridden preoccupations. They then need individual help in facing the difficulties of the new situation after hidden conflicts have been forced into the open. I have seen schizophrenic patients regress after such conferences because they felt overpowered by the openly revealed evidence of hatred and deep misunderstandings, and by their conviction of helplessness to do anything about it.

Work with a patient's family is important and exceedingly useful if handled skillfully and tactfully. Treating a patient in the hospital and sending him back into a family where nothing has changed is an outdated practice, apt to result in a relapse. Not involving the family in the therapeutic process often leads to premature interruption of treatment, not uncommonly at the point where a patient just begins to change and shows it by becoming more self-assertive. Excluded relatives will experience increasing tension and discontent when the delicate balance that kept them going before the patient became sick begins to change.

I recall the case of Karl, a young man who became psychotic during his first year in college and whose family reacted with sacrificing but hopeless despair. There were voluble expressions of gratitude when Karl was well enough to return to college. Treatment was continued on an out-patient basis, but there were increasing complaints about the length of treatment and the son's not being respectful enough. The patient felt that he had never been able to talk freely to his father, who was absorbed in his busy law practice. They had become even more estranged because Karl would not consider law as a career and refused to study the courses his father thought important. It appeared to be a promising step when the father requested to see the therapist—Karl hoped that his father had finally recognized the need for greater closeness. When the father came it was only to inform the patient and the therapist that he no longer felt legally responsible to pay for treatment since the therapist supported his son's career plan, of which he disapproved, and since Karl was going to be twenty-one years old.

This painful confrontation could have been avoided if there had been more constructive contact with the family. With some clarification of the son's need for genuine independence, the father reconsidered his stand and treatment was continued. The episode became an important turning point in the therapy: it showed the extent to which Karl had made his own moving ahead, and the development of trust in his growing maturity, dependent on the father's participation.

The need for integrating work with the family into the therapeutic effort was first recognized in the treatment of children, and it has been increasingly extended to the treatment of adolescents and young adults. However, there is no *one* way that would be best for effecting changes in the interactions and emotional climate of the home, one that would be applicable to all families. Interviews with the family should be conducted so that something constructive can be achieved for each member; they should not be accusatory and guilt-provoking. This is of particular importance when dealing with families in which blame transfer had been the dominant way of mutual interaction. Though a patient's illness can clearly be traced to faulty and harmful relations within the family, it must be remembered that the others only rarely acted in a deliberately malicious way. Usually the others were also motivated by unresolved and unrecognized conflicts and handicaps. It is important to show consideration and respect for the relatives who may be unhappy and insecure, however outrageously and unreasonably we feel the patient has been treated. In child psychiatry parents often look upon the therapist as an enemy. Unavoidably parents feel defensive about the very fact that a child is in treatment; it is an admission of failure. But mutual hostility may be related to the therapist's overidentifying with his child-patient, and to his critical and reproachful attitude toward the parents.

In the face of psychiatric illness, families tend to feel under attack. They project onto the psychiatrist their sense of failure and their resentment that the need for psychiatric treatment makes this public. Such families may have great talent in denying all problems and will give a distorted and overoptimistic picture of what has gone on. They will disclaim the existence even of desperate illness in one of them, and suffer at the prospect that some skeleton in the closet will be exposed; the whole structure of the family interaction had been centered on making things appear different from what they really were. The fact of overt mental illness only adds to the list of what must be kept secret. A conference with a family may be arranged in the hope of getting a more realistic picture, but it must be kept in mind that it may not turn out as revealing as had been expected, and that the family's misrepresentations may add to the confusion.

FAMILY INTERFERENCE

Still, even misunderstandings, or what looks like unnecessary "interference," may at times lead to clarification of what has been going on. Angela was a young married woman who had become severely depressed and was in such an extreme state of tension that hospitalization became necessary, early in December. After she had quieted down somewhat, she began to plead for permission to spend the approaching holidays with her parents, who lived in a different part of the country. Since so little was known about her and her background, she and her husband were advised to postpone the visit until something therapeutically useful could be gained from it. The parents were given the same explanation but refused to accept it, and an endless number of letters and telephone calls ensued. When the excitement was at its height, Angela suddenly declared that a visit home at this time would be wrong. She had dreamed that, as she tried to enter her parents' house, her old cat hissed furiously at her to keep her from entering. This meant to her that her place was now with her husband, no longer with her parents.

A comment was made that the dream also suggested that not everything in her parents' home was sweetness and light, as she had claimed. She agreed that there were unresolved conflicts but would not enlarge on the topic.

A week or two later her father became highly indignant when he could not reach the therapist by phone, to discuss another visit. He went up the line of command until he finally reached the head of the service about his having been ignored. When this episode was taken up in therapy, in particular the father's impatient complaining to the higher authority, Angela opened up and explained that this had always been the real trouble with her father, that his feelings were easily hurt. Even as a child she thought she must devote her whole life to protecting him against anything he might deem hurtful; in particular, she had felt obliged to be "perfect" to save him any pain or disappointment.

The father found many more reasons to ask for special consideration. Angela finally wrote, begging him to postpone a visit until she had a clearer understanding of what had caused her desperate depression and panic. The fact that the father repeatedly put the therapist in the position of having to say "no" became an important topic in therapy; the patient reexperienced how she had always felt pressured into complete submission. Though her brothers had rebelled at times, she had never dared refuse anything her father demanded. (The way in which Angela freed herself from this unquestioning submission will be discussed in Chapter Seven.)

ALOOFNESS FROM THE FAMILY

Staying completely away from a patient's family, particularly when blatantly abnormal behavior is apparent, may result in therapeutic stalemate and progressive deterioration of a patient's whole life. This is apt to happen when a patient's symptoms arouse a great deal of anxiety in others; as time goes on, this usually changes to resentment and anger. Families do not dare express their feelings or act on them, because the patient uses his even greater anger to coerce them to give in to him, by suicidal threats or dramatic display of anxiety states. Whatever the psychological constellation that precipitated an illness, as the condition persists symptoms tend to lose their original dynamic meaning; but they acquire an interpersonal significance and are used for coercive purposes. Phobic states may lead to such self-perpetuating stalemates, and the patient becomes increasingly more articulate in describing his states of terror and panic, with threats of dire consequences. Such a patient will quietly go about his life as long as the designated "collaborator" does exactly as told. Symptoms may persist over the years, though the dynamics have been thoroughly explained. When the total situation is explored in a consultation, one may find that the therapist and a relative had been competing to see who was better at allaying the anxiety. When the Gordian knot is cut by exposing the ongoing interpersonal issues, the phobia, though of long duration, often dissolves.

In other conditions, too, where a patient's threats and demands for immediate fulfillment have a paralyzing influence on the family, similar entanglements may stymie all therapeutic efforts. One obese girl "dieted" by forcing her parents to shop three times a day because she would not permit any food in the home between meals. Everything left over had to be thrown away because she feared that she might succumb to the compulsion of eating. She became physically aggressive and created violent scenes when she gained as little as an ounce. The parents put up with this because their daughter's psychiatrist had implored them to be patient. He himself complied with the girl's demand that he should never mention the word *food,* and he urged the parents to obey her and never to talk about food. In another case the father of an anorexic girl, a well-known business tycoon, confessed, "We are completely buffaloed—but her doctor told us to go along with her"; he had rearranged his home, building a special kitchen for the daughter where she would cook all night. Needless to say, the anorexic condition had not improved in spite of the girl's having been in therapy for over five years, and there were manifestations of increasing anxiety, depression, and withdrawal.

HOSPITALIZATION

The orthodox analytic rule of strictly separating therapy and other aspects of living has also been applied to hospitalized patients. Psychiatric hospitals with this philosophy will divide the care for a patient between two therapists: one who functions as psychotherapist and the other, as administrator, who will make the day-by-day decisions about the practical aspects of a patient's life. In other hospitals, and this is the more common arrangement, the psychotherapist is also responsible for the range of "privileges" and activities of his patients. Although it may avoid certain problems, the separation into therapeutic and administrative components can create new difficulties, which interfere with progress when they remain hidden and unacknowledged. There may be disagreement between the therapist and administrator, with one viewing the other as "too indulgent" or "too punitive." Patients are apt to respond to tension between the people on whom they are dependent with a relapse, or with the development of new symptoms. The isolation of the therapeutic relationship from the other realities of a patient's life also carries the danger, particularly in extremely dependent or schizophrenic patients, that the therapist-patient relationship will become too exclusive and precious: it may thus reenact distortions in the early mother-child relationship to which much of the maldevelopment can be traced.

Student therapists have a tendency to side with the patient

against all kinds of hospital routine as too arbitrary or too restrictive. Today a patient's role is conceived of as much more active, and there has been a considerable decrease of such restrictions. In such an improved and liberalized therapeutic climate, situations will come up where an individual patient may need special supervision or restriction of his activities. Disentanglement of the underlying unconscious knots and distortions continues to be the essential task of psychotherapy, and there are many situations where familiarity with these inner problems enables the therapist to help with the practical aspects of a patient's daily life; at times he may have to give direct advice. Even sophisticated patients are at times glaringly uninformed about certain commonsense aspects of living, and then the therapist may be called upon to function as an educator.

Instead of interfering with therapeutic progress, attention to the immediate aspects of living, physical complaints, difficulties with hospital routine, disturbances on the ward, and so forth, offers important raw material for psychotherapeutic investigation. If therapy under these conditions deteriorates into a power struggle between patient and therapist, I am inclined to explore the problems of the physician who cannot handle it or who does not remain objective in the face of such complexities. There are some exceptions to the management of all aspects of a patient's care by only one person, such as psychosomatic disorders where the management of the physical condition should be left to a medical specialist. However, the problems that come up in connection with this are legitimate material for the psychotherapeutic inquiry.

The greater range of activities in a modern hospital and the encouraged interaction with other patients offer valuable material to be discussed and explored in individual therapeutic sessions. As new treatment modalities were being introduced, there was in the beginning some debate whether a patient in individual psychotherapy should also attend group meetings or be in group therapy. Now that the dust has settled, it appears that involvement with many different people enlivens and broadens what comes up during individual sessions, and adds considerably to a patient's chances of recovery.

In terms of staff interaction, patients are sensitive to tensions and disagreements between different people on the hospital staff, and may react with new symptoms or even ask to be discharged when they feel caught between the conflicting attitudes and contradictory messages or when open rivalry leads to a lack of respect for the other's point of view. Fred, a young man of nineteen, requested a consultation to gain reassurance that he had not thrown away his chance of recovery by leaving a residential treatment center against medical advice. Before hospitalization his behavior had been quite unmanageable, with uncontrollable temper outbursts and violent, often bizarre attacks on various members of his family. He had made good progress during a year of treatment but became upset when his first therapist, whom he greatly admired, left the service and a fellow patient, a young woman to whom he had been closely attached, was discharged. He had never been able to tolerate a personal loss without acute depression or compensatory rages. The new therapist, instead of helping Fred with his grief reaction, began to attack the previous therapist for having permitted too close a relationship to develop and for not having explored the symbolic meaning of certain symptoms; in this way "a whole year of treatment had been lost." Fred decided to leave because he felt that this belittling criticism of his former therapist undermined something of value to him. The impulsiveness of his reaction suggested that not all had been well in the previous therapeutic relationship. But whatever correction needed to be made, it was handled so that the patient experienced it as destructive, as if the new therapist were presenting himself as more "analytical' and superior in his approach.

Patients are also quite aware of the status and prestige of the various therapists, and they will test out whether a low rank in the pecking order interferes with a therapist's usefulness. This was vividly brought home to me quite early in my residency. Anna, a thirty-six-year-old woman and a former nun, was assigned to me as one of my first patients. She had been an invalid for the past eight years and suffered from such a variety of symptoms that she referred to them as "too numerous to mention and told as often as Mother Goose rhymes." She had been in nearly continuous medical and psychiatric treatment, with several hospitalizations, and was deeply attached to the referring psychiatrist. She was overfriendly toward me, but in a condescending way since it was quite obvious that she was much more of an expert than I could ever hope to be. Assignment to the latest newcomer was to her a reflection of her own low status, that she was considered unworthy of an experienced therapist. She made a good adjustment to the ward where she felt at home, having been a former patient at the clinic, and superficially she appeared cooperative. In spite of her "wanting to cooperate," she resisted attending activities or following other routines, as too upsetting and exhausting. Though no pressure was used to make her conform, she became very agitated, developing a coarse tremor, at times so severe that she was unable to stand up. She was equally disturbed when she forced herself to participate in activities.

During the second week of her stay, an incident occurred which appeared out of character with her apparent meekness. Anna flatly refused to be interviewed by a medical student, an accepted routine in a teaching hospital, stuck vehemently to this decision, and became quite rude. She explained that her refusal had nothing to do with the medical student as a person, that she had decided before she had ever seen him. When her reasons for this behavior were explored, she expressed surprise that there were no disciplinary consequences. The leniency in regard to her nonparticipation in activities had not been convincing; she had been living in constant dread of being punished for breaking the rules. She wanted to prove her ability *not* to be forced to do what she had decided not to do, and also to test the "courage" of her new therapist. Refusing to be interviewed by a medical student meant defying several people in the clinic's hierarchy; she wanted to find out how far her inexperienced therapist would back her up, though it might mean trouble for herself. Much material relating to the destructive significance of "obedience" in her life subsequently came into the open. Being forced to obey had played a significant role in the development of her illness, and she felt she was not worthy of special effort on her behalf. Anna made a surprisingly good recovery; some of the significant steps will be discussed later (Chapter Seven).

Other patients may be more direct, even crudely assaultive, in their belittling of a new therapist, usually with unfavorable comparison to a previous therapist. This is apt to happen when there is growing intimacy and good progress in a therapeutic relationship, which is then interrupted because the therapist, at the end of his training, must leave the service. When skillfully handled, as a regrettable but unavoidable life event, and with an open-minded and constructive evaluation of what has been achieved so far and what problems have been left untouched, such a change, though on the whole undesirable, may be used constructively. Quite often it offers a chance to bring out aspects of the therapeutic interaction that had remained obscure to the patient, and also at times to the former therapist. Many other administrative problems and misunderstandings come up and offer helpful material for psychotherapeutic exploration.

MEDICATION

The introduction of tranquilizers and other psychotropic drugs has broadened the field for psychotherapy, but it has also introduced new complications that need to be considered in the context of each individual situation. Psychotherapy was an effective treatment method before drugs were available to modify the devastating and disintegrating effects of panic and pervasive anxiety. The early therapists felt able to allay anxiety through skillful intervention. There are still some who reject the modifying influence of all medication under the credo that in order to become a truly integrated person, with full insight into his problems, a patient needs to understand the sources of his anxiety, work through the issues that precipitate it, and recognize his capacity to tolerate stress. Some have expressed concern whether "learning," which is part of all psychotherapy, can be effective and enduring if a patient was under the influence of drugs when it took place. At the other extreme, overenthusiastic advertising has made it appear that the new drugs have solved the problems of mental illness and that they have raised psychiatry to the level of a "medical" speciality. Neither claim is entirely correct.

Provided drugs are not used in dosages that completely obliterate a person's awareness of his problems and transform him into a zombie, they are valuable adjuncts to psychotherapy and allow previously inaccessible patients, such as disorganized schizophrenics, to engage more easily in a helpful therapeutic relationship. In particular, they permit treatment in a time perspective that is more realistic in the patient's total life cycle than the timeless devotion reflected in the early reports on the psychotherapy of schizophrenia.

Some young psychiatrists are so dependent on psychotropic drugs that they have drawn the conclusion that treatment without them would be impossible, or would involve unbearable hardship for patients. The few brief sketches given here of treatment of patients during my own residency, when psychotropic drugs were not yet available, will serve to demonstrate that effective treatment is possible, and without undue demands on a patient's endurance, through psychotherapeutic intervention alone. When agitated or upset, these patients were given traditional sedatives. At that time electroshock had just come into use. It was propagated as a cureall for schizophrenia and everything else, with the same uncritical enthusiasm with which the psychotropic drugs are touted today.

On the whole, a judicious balance has begun to develop between the use of drugs and psychotherapy, though some recent graduates use drugs with such matter-of-factness, or resort to them whenever the going gets rough, that they are unaware they are denying their conviction that psychotherapy can be effective. On the other side, some die-hard psychotherapists of the old school feel that "giving" anything to a patient will interfere with the therapeutic relationship, or reinforce a patient's dependency, or result in transforming the image of the therapist into that of a magician. There is no doubt that tranquilizers are useful in severe anxiety states, depression, and periods of disorganization, and it is also a fact that some patients will interpret the receiving of a drug as a magical act. This becomes a problem if the therapist is not aware of it, or if he does indeed behave like a magician. Prescribing a tranquilizer or antidepressant without awareness that this introduces new parameters into the therapeutic field may result in a grave distortion of the therapeutic interaction, whereas a clear awareness of the situation can render psychotropic drugs useful and may shorten treatment time. The important point is that they should not be offered as a substitute for a meaningful therapeutic relationship. Although drugs have an ameliorating effect on the most disturbing and destructive symptoms, they do not improve or correct the underlying symbolic deficits and distorted life experiences.

Even when the therapist has these ideas in mind, the patient may experience receiving medication in many different ways, and the issues must be explored openly in therapy. He may come to feel that the physician "controls" him through the pills, and an anxious therapist may be doing exactly that and may feel that his own functioning is dependent on the pills. Others feel that all the talking, reporting of fantasies and dreams, and such, is empty words, the price you have to pay to get a prescription, that the pills are the real treatment. It may also be experienced as an admission of defeat, that the therapist does not truly believe in the effectiveness of the therapeutic interaction. Such interpretations are not always incorrect. There are therapists who feel at a loss without prescribing something, and patients may observe this when the therapist is insecure about establishing or maintaining the relationship.

The more immature and dependent a patient, the more likely he will conceive of a prescription as standing symbolically for a psychological gift. He has entered therapy with the expectation that the therapist will give him something special and convey to him qualities that will result in his cure, through an increase in self-confidence and power, maturity and independence. Such fantasies and misperceptions must be brought into the open, and the patient needs help in understanding that, though he has the capacity to acquire all these desirable qualities, he can do it only through active participation in therapy, through his own growth and development.

4

The Patient Speaks

Psychoanalysis has been called the "talking cure," and exchange of words has remained the most obvious form of communication in psychotherapy. The reality of the therapeutic involvement is far more than simply verbal, however, and much more than an exchange of words and information takes place.

FEARS AND EXPECTATIONS

Psychiatric patients differ greatly not only in the complaints that bring them to your office, but in their education, cultural background, and concepts of what psychiatry is all about. Old fears and prejudices that psychiatry deals with crazy people linger on, as well as notions that it is shameful to admit needing help with personal problems or that one's illness is not real but reveals a weakness for which one has only himself to blame.

A negative attitude with openly expressed doubts about needing psychiatric help, or about the value of psychiatry, is not incompatible with a good treatment result. As a matter of fact, I find it more amenable to successful intervention than overenthusiastic expressions of faith in psychiatry or in the therapist. Of course, a rigid inability for introspective reporting, or absolute refusal to do so, will make it hard, if not impossible, to clarify the underlying psychological issues. This type of extreme negativism becomes a problem in the treatment of involuntary patients who have been committed to a treatment center, or when a patient considers his symptoms actually desirable. In anorexia nervosa patients will insist that nothing is wrong, that they are "not too thin"; on the contrary they live in dread of becoming too fat. Others may vigorously object to psychiatric treatment though they submit to it in martyr fashion.

Every patient comes with an attitude in which realistic expectations are mixed with irrational elements. It is the specific task of psychotherapy to expose and correct the irrational factors, even those that are part of the general cultural attitude, because unexplored they might becloud the treatment progress. Though aware that psychotherapy is different from ordinary medical treatment, patients will endow the therapist with the same qualities with which our culture endows the physician, namely special knowledge, prestige, authority, and help-giving ability. People turn to psychotherapy for help with the problems of living they cannot manage alone. It is the desire to be free of insecurities, helplessness, and loneliness, a tendency toward health, that brings one to a therapist, and keeps him coming. This hope and desire for help is important in the bond that develops between therapist and patient, and it will develop regardless of the therapist's professional or chronological age.

The patient needs to discover that nothing is "given" to him, that therapy is a process which involves the active acquisition of self-understanding. To accomplish this he must learn to mobilize his own resources and develop his potentialities. It is important to clarify early in treatment a patient's concepts of "psychiatric help," and this may need repeated reformulation until he grasps that he really has the ability to be an active participant in the therapeutic process, though the hope may linger on that he will receive all the desirable qualities—self-confidence, popularity, sexual prowess, attractiveness, and so on—from the therapist.

Particular problems are encountered in the treatment of those who appear sophisticated and are quite articulate in expressing that they know what psychotherapy is about, those who usually are rated as well-motivated, cooperative, and good prospects for successful therapy. Such a patient may nevertheless indulge in the fantasy that there is a right formula and answer to his problem, and that one of these days, as a reward for good behavior, the therapist will reveal it to him and thus cure him. Even people who by virtue of their professional position or education are expected to be well informed may proceed with an attitude of "I'll tell you everything and then you'll know what's the matter with me and can tell me what to do." Not uncommonly, if this issue has not been clarified, disappointment leads to growing resentment and sullen, barely disguised hostility, which arise from the feeling of "you are not giving me what I expect and what is due me," or "you are withholding from me what you know." The patient's seeming familiarity with psychoanalytic terminology should not be interpreted as indicating that he is not in need of such basic clarification of treatment goals. Regardless of what the therapist understands or sees in a different light, the patient will learn to view his life in a new perspective only by uncovering all the ramifications of what is bothering him. In this way he also develops the mental tools to do something concrete about his difficulties.

Therapeutic exploration involves detailed discussion of the most private aspects of one's life. Most patients, though by no means all, are to some extent prepared for this, but they may nevertheless consider self-revelation as a painful invasion of, or relentless intrusion into, their privacy. The youngster who explained to a friend, "A psychiatrist is a guy who makes you squeal on yourself," expressed succinctly what many others have felt. Most are well enough informed to accept that they will have to reveal their sexual practices and fantasies, and will do so with a certain determined courage to "tell it all." Many find it much more difficult to reveal seemingly trivial topics, such as embarrassment about one's body and its deviation from perfection, admission of petty jealousies, envy, or dishonesties, snobbish attitudes about one's social position, or embarrassment about one's uncultured background. Much of what appears as resistance often is a quite conscious concern not to appear in a lesser light than one had first presented oneself, nor to permit a glimpse behind the facade so carefully constructed to cover up for an underlying fear of worthlessness.

For such a patient the hardest rule to follow is simply to be honest. Some obsessives will go to great lengths to keep the true facts concealed, to omit what they declare to be irrelevancies, to distort in the next sentence what they have just said in the last, or to reverse themselves from one session to another, all in an exaggerated effort to keep up appearances. To them the treatment process is not a common enterprise, an alliance, but an adversary process in which the important goal is "to win," to outsmart the therapist who is "the enemy." This, of course, is no longer a conscious attitude but the outcome of life-long processes brought into the treatment relationship.

Patients are influenced in their expectations about therapy through what they have heard or read, or on the basis of a previous treatment experience. Someone who speaks "expertly" about his complexes, about the "Oedipus bit" or "anal stuff," or who constantly talks about having trouble with "authority figures," is unlikely to reveal his real feelings as he experiences them with people in his life or with the therapist. Others are more direct in expressing distrust or hostility which they claim had been created by previous professional contacts.

PREVIOUS THERAPY

I should like to give an example of a patient who brought his previous treatment experiences unexamined into the new relationship. Jim, a twenty-eight-year-old man who had suffered a psychotic episode ten years earlier, came to me for additional treatment after moving from a different city to New York. He felt unable to put real effort into his work, had difficulties with his fellow workers and also in his marriage. He described his former treatment experience as enjoyable; he had been involved in what he thought of as friendly competition with his analyst, namely which one could discover first the symbolic meaning of Jim's long dreams and copious associations. Even now he would spend many hours thinking about his dreams, and he felt that this interferred with completing his Ph.D. thesis.

He felt that the relationship had been warm and friendly, with no overt expression of angry feelings, though he had always been late and thought this had been his way of showing hostility. I expressed the hope that he would make full use of his treatment time now and would feel free to be more direct in expressing his feelings. To his own amazement Jim was on time for appointments. One day, twenty minutes after the scheduled time, the doorbell rang frantically. Jim's face was flushed and staring at his watch he said accusingly, "You kept me waiting twenty minutes, I am not going to change the time." In the past his anger would have been unacceptable and he would have become unclear about the time, saying that maybe he had misread his watch. He accepted an apology for having been kept waiting. Then he admitted that he was already upset on arrival because he was late, though unintentionally; sure this would be interpreted as "hostile," he had rung the doorbell quite softly at first. The door to my office was ajar and he heard the sound of talking, which then stopped and which he correctly interpreted as the end of a telephone conversation. When he was not asked into the office immediately, he became terribly enraged because he felt I was punishing him for being hostile.

It was a real revelation for Jim to learn that there are mishaps without sinister meaning, and that the sequence of events could be elucidated by a simple factual account of what had happened. I had noticed before that Jim tended to draw immediate, and often unjustified, motivational conclusions, but repeated discussions had been ineffective until then. It had been recognized that his nearly automatic investing of even the smallest mishap with some emotional significance was related to a psychologizing mother, who never accepted a fact as a fact but always gave it some hidden, usually malevolent interpretation. To a lesser degree it was related to his previous treatment experience, but the tendency had remained unexamined. He recognized now for the first time how his motivational "interpretations" interfered with his taking effective action, and had also led to many altercations between him and his co-workers. He had never understood how other people would know the difference between intentional behavior and accidental events. During this careful evaluation Jim felt for the first time that he was an active participant in the treatment process, that he understood what had happened, and that his role was not just one of waiting for the boom to come down to reveal him again as incompetent or hostile.

STYLE OF COMMUNICATION

Attention to the style in which a patient speaks about himself may add an extra dimension to the understanding of his problems. Bart, a patient who had always been close to his mother, had come to recognize his resentment of her intrusion into every aspect of his life. In spite of much talk of his anger and rage, with displays of seemingly appropriate emotion, there was no real change. When speaking of upsetting memories or current quarrels with his mother, he would say in a plaintive voice, "Then something happened to me," and go on to describe his reaction. After this mannerism of using the passive form had been pointed out, without discussion of what the "something" was, he began to recognize that in this way he had indirectly disclaimed responsibility for the feelings he had described so vividly, often exaggeratedly, and thus he could cling to the delusion of being a sweet, helpless boy who himself could not really experience such vulgar emotions. Only after acknowledging such feelings as his own did Bart really progress and mature.

Another example is that of Greta, who at the age of fifteen had developed anorexia nervosa, of which she said later, "This was the only way to fight back." She summarized her background: "My mother overprotected me psychologically, and my father spoiled me materialistically." With good medical care and supportive psychiatric treatment she regained weight and finished high school. Greta wanted to become an actress, but whenever she had a chance to take part in a play she had episodes of depression and compulsive eating. Acting to her was the fulfillment of exhibitionistic fantasies, of being a cute little girl on the stage, admired and applauded by everyone but chiefly by her parents. She recognized the need for training and entered drama school, where she did fairly well. Yet she would resort to eating binges after the slightest criticism, with the complaint, "I work as hard as anybody, without getting the benefit from it." This was rephrased to her one day as, "In other words, you do not perform as well as you expect?" Greta was silent for a time and then asked, "You mean we can't blame it all on my parents?" She began to recognize her self-image as the completely passive product of her parents' doings and her craving for admiration and praise as a means of assuring her success.

By paying attention to the way language is used, the therapist can convey to a patient, in an indirect way, in the day-by-day interaction, that he is a person capable of experiencing his own thoughts, feelings, and sensations, and not an inert mouthpiece, repeating only what others have told him to think or feel. This amounts to a close collaborative examination of a patient's inner resources and potentiality for development. The fact that he is being *listened to,* and *not told by someone else* what he really feels or means, is in itself an important new experience—that he and what comes from him are worthwhile.

Sometimes the acknowledgment of the feeling that the therapist is tuned in correcly takes a dramatic form. An eighteen-year-old girl, Tanya, needed help with her deep sense of isolation and was exceedingly vague and noncommital in talking about herself. However, she was quite outspoken and sarcastic in tearing others down; her particular objects of attack were psychiatrists and clergymen because, though revered as having everything figured out, they seemed to have troubles of their own: "If they are not perfect, what right have they to superimpose their opinions on others?" Once as Tanya was rambling on with gossip about some psychiatrists, I drew her attention to certain contradictions in what she was saying. She burst out crying, an emotional response quite out of the proportion to the apparent levity of her facetious remarks. As I was wondering what in my comment had hit a sensitive spot, she gave the explanation, *"But you listened, you listened!"* Her tears were tears of relief that something new had happened; I had carefully listened even to her trivial and catty remarks. The feeling of loneliness from which Tanya had suffered even as a child was related to never having had the feeling that her parents listened to her. Father was too busy and important, interested in great things only. Mother said she wanted to know everything that went on in her daughter's life, but then never noticed when she was told things that were nonsensical or contradictory. It was out of these experiences, or at least what they represented to her, that Tanya had come to the conviction that grown-ups were not really interested in children and that children were made to do things according to the grown-ups' whims without consideration for what they really needed. She had gone through life convinced that whatever she did, or was expected to do, was forced upon her and that none of her activities was in any form related to her own life.

Following this episode Tanya revealed bit by bit some of the absorbing fantasies with which she had entertained herself, preferring them to companionship with young people, which made her appear severely withdrawn. "I have two worlds, and the better world is the dream world. I am always a little in it and hate to be interrupted; but one can always pretend. When you listened to me, I was completely out of the dream world nobody approves of. The real world is solid and things stay put, and the two together are liquid and things change."

NONVERBAL COMMUNICATION

In psychotherapy, as in any other human contact, there is much more to communication than words. The simple fact of meeting regularly and spending time together in the same room may be as significant an expression of a definite commitment, even more so, as whether a patient talks, is silent or sullen, asks questions, smiles, or weeps. However much a patient objects to needing psychiatry, or criticizes the therapist, keeping his appointments indicates that some bond is developing, along with an implied expectation and hope for understanding.

Sometimes articulate patients will use words to hide things— or to keep the therapist from inquiring and finding out the hidden meanings. Silences may be more communicative; often they are a plea for understanding. *How* something is said may change the meaning of *what* has been said; throughout our lives we have always known that to understand a message one must read between the lines. In listening to a patient, watching for some relevant gesture and expression is as important as hearing the words. As Freud expressed it: "He that has eyes to see and ears to hear may convince himself that no mortal can keep a secret. If his lips are silent, he chatters with his fingertips, betrayal oozes out of him at every pore."

In recent years the importance of nonverbal communication has become the object for serious scientific study, and we all have become more aware of its significance in expressing important aspects of interpersonal relationships. Hopelessness and despair may be expressed more clearly in posture or gesture or tone of voice than in any specific words; or a conforming statement may be expressed in a defiant tone or be accompanied by clenched hands. The full message will not be grasped without attention to changing gestures, huskiness or fullness of voice, blushing or slight stiffening that accompanies the words. These indirect messages may give important clues about the significant areas to be explored. In addition, probably nothing demonstrates more convincingly that therapeutic communication is a two-way process than the therapist's own nonverbal cues, which the patient interprets in his way and which may tell him whether his doctor is relaxed and attentive or tense, bewildered, and even bored.

Sometimes a patient himself may draw attention to the meaning of his gestures. Peter, a bright student, entered treatment because he was having great difficulty in finishing his thesis and he expressed bitter resentment about having to fulfill so many unnecessary requirements. He was reluctant to express feelings about therapy, or to admit having any particular feelings, until he noted that he had a habit of crossing his legs and that this occurred when he slowed down in talking or stopped altogether. He recognized its significance, a desire to "hold in," not to let things come out too freely, out of fear that he might be giving "ammunition to the enemy." Peter had a habit of making current events "history," keeping notes on his activities and even getting up at night to dictate into a tape recorder, with the explanation that he couldn't trust his memory. Actually he was afraid that something would "give him away" if he talked spontaneously. When his intellectualized reporting had been pointed out to him before, he had felt attacked. After he had recognized the meaning of the leg-crossing gesture, he began to express ideas and feelings as they occurred to him, regardless of their implications.

There are many indirect ways in which therapist and patient communicate how they think and feel about each other. Even being accepted for therapy may be a discouraging message; it confirms the fear that there is "something the matter with me," dashing the hope to be declared normal and not in need of treatment. Others feel the opposite, that the therapist does not recognize how sick they really are and does not see them often enough. Still others feel disappointed that they are not on the couch—only that would be real treatment—or, the reverse, the possibility of being on the couch arouses alarm.

There are other hidden ways through which a patient communicates what troubles him, though it may not be expressed directly in the therapeutic sessions. Dave was a graduate student who came for treatment because he alternated between compulsive and exhausting absorption in his work and complete indifference. He was in conflict about his career, which he felt he pursued in order to satisfy his father who had died suddenly just at the time of the decision to enter graduate school. He felt obliged to follow his father's career in spite of serious doubts and lack of motivation. He had been well provided for financially so that he did not even have the challenge of having to earn his livelihood.

Though obviously involved in treatment and eager to progress, Dave was repeatedly late for his sessions, with vague and irritated explanations about parking difficulties. A few days after he had finally decided to pursue a career of his own choosing, he appeared on time, was relaxed and looked relieved. He confessed that he had solved another dilemma. Among other things, Dave had "inherited" his father's big black limousine; he had felt it acutely embarrassing for a student to drive such a conspicuous car, but he could not dispose of it since it had come to him from his father. After he had recognized the unreasonable degree of attachment to his dead father, he finally took the step of selling the big monster and bought a small car, appropriate to his student status and no longer advertising that he was an "heir."

DREAMS

Beginning therapists are often reluctant to make use of dreams because it might imply that they are "doing psychoanalysis." Most have some vague knowledge that the manifest dream content does not count, that only "analysis" reveals the true meaning, the hidden unconscious content, and in order to get at it a patient must "associate" to every word. In the classical model, dreams were considered "the royal road to the unconscious"; like everything else in psychoanalysis, the place and interpretation of dreams have changed considerably.

Whatever one's theoretical concepts, dreams do make an important contribution to the understanding of what troubles people, particularly in those who hesitate to reveal themselves or are otherwise inhibited in exploring their underlying thoughts and feelings. As unconscious communication, dreams are guideposts to hidden problems that preoccupy an individual but have been avoided or are not readily accessible. They are particularly useful in working with patients who feel that everything is being imposed upon them from the outside, that what they feel and think does not count: one can stress that dreams originate in the patient and through them he reveals in his own imagery how he experiences himself or the world around him.

One young woman, Sharon, denied, in spite of many serious difficulties, that there were any underlying problems or diffi-

culties with her family. She felt that she did not really need intensive treatment, until she dreamed about their summer home of
which she had reported only pleasant memories. There was a
railed balcony on the third floor which was quite high up and
overlooked the garden, but in the dream instead of a garden
there was water below. On the rail there was a man, hanging by
one hand, and she knew instinctively that he was "bad." The
idea was to get rid of him by making him fall from the balcony
into the water below. Someone was pulling this bad man by one
leg and someone strong, a faceless person, was pounding his hand
with a pail until he finally fell off. Sharon herself now had to
undergo the test and was hanging from the balcony, then
dropped from the rail and sank beneath the water. She suddenly
realized that she could not breathe and woke with a start in a
panic.

This frightening dream in a way gave Sharon permission to
talk about the not so perfect aspects of her life, the precarious-
ness of her own position and her futile efforts to maintain the
fictitious image of perfection, her helplessness in relation to
others. One can, of course, interpret dreams in many different
ways; I am offering various aspects here to show the usefulness
of the *process* in having patients deal with the frightening problems of living in more open ways.

Sometimes a dream will reveal in a startling image a patient's
helpless struggle with ill-defined urges. In one such instance a
graduate student, concerned about dropping out because he felt
dissatisfied and uncommitted to his professional choice, dreamed
that he was thirsty, went to the refrigerator, and drank some
milk. He was still thirsty and drank some more but, however
much he drank, he remained thirsty. He woke up feeling thirsty
but did not dare drink because he felt that whatever he drank
would not quench his thirst. Following this dream he began to
examine the emotional aspects of his personal life which inter-

fered with his ability to experience satisfaction, instead of ruminating about his future profession and whether it would satisfy him or not.

At times a dream may reveal a patient's concept of what is going on in relation to treatment. In an eighteen-year-old girl who had been severely depressed, her repetitious statements of "It is useless" were recognized as relating to the critical attitude of her parents toward her need for treatment. She dreamed that she had suffered an injury and her leg was in a cast that was falling into pieces, tearing away the shriveled-up skin and muscles and exposing the bone. Nobody seemed to care but kept urging her, "Come on, come on," and she had to go about her business whether she was able to or not. Within a month treatment was discontinued by the family as "no longer necessary." Needless to say, she relapsed and became suicidal.

A dream may also express the opposite and foreshadow the possibility of a more satisfactory life. After many years of unsuccessful treatment efforts, a young woman showed the first signs of improvement. She dreamed that she was in an Alpine meadow, carrying a child on her arm and passing by huts, exchanging friendly greetings with the mountain people. She was still so doubting that she wanted to dismiss this dream as ridiculous and was rather annoyed when it was pointed out to her that she seemed to have some inner awareness, despite all her protestations to the contrary, of her capacities for a happier life. Years later, after a good recovery and after she married and had children, she confessed that in spite of all her negative remarks, this dream had stayed in her mind and sustained her in periods of despair.

Sometimes certain dream images appear repeatedly, but with variations that reflect changes as treatment progresses. Claire, a graduate student of twenty-four who obtained her Ph.D. while in treatment in spite of the seriousness of her problems, dreamed over and over that she was in an elevator. At first she was all alone and the elevator would go out of control and explode, or go through the roof, or lead to some other disaster. As she improved the elevator dreams continued, but she was no longer alone—people entered and left on different floors, and finally she too reached the correct floor and her destination.

Claire, though ambulatory and capable of functioning in certain areas, expressed herself in startling symbols whenever she was confused in her thinking. She came for treatment with complaints about being depressed, that she slept poorly and was unable to concentrate; continuous fatigue was her most disturbing symptom. She had been married for one year but felt disappointed because her marriage was not perfect, and she worried about being unwanted and unloved. She appeared on the point of disorganization and tranquilizers were prescribed. This became to her a sign that the physician was "in control" and that it was the pills that kept her going. She tried to keep the therapist in the position of being in control by waiting for him to ask questions, with the air of "you show me" and by insisting that she herself had nothing to say. If the therapist made a comment that seemed relevant, particularly if it concerned other people, the patient deducted that he had some special magic or was a mindreader.

Claire gradually mentioned some of her peculiar habits. Even before coming for treatment she had suffered, at times of upheaval and decision making, episodes she called "psycho-sick." At one time she thought she was dead, lay on the floor and could not move. At other times she would get strong feelings of wanting to hide, would go to the bathroom and squeeze between the toilet and the wall, or she might crawl into the knee hole of her husband's desk. She would spend as much as an hour or longer in such narrow corners. She explained that in order to think she had to be "out of the open spaces" and therefore sought a confined hideaway. All this she would report in a matter-of-fact way, as natural behavior.

When upset, and this might follow upon any argument, be it in class, at the lab, even on TV, and whether it involved her or not, Claire would experience a whirling sensation, with her head spinning around. She had the feeling that her husband could read her mind; she felt that people passing in their car who looked at her knew what she was thinking. Her hair had come to be symbolic of herself. When somebody criticized the way her hair looked she would feel severely censured, as if it were a personal attack. "If my hair is messed up, so is my mind."

In therapy the focus was on her fear of not having autonomy and control, which she expressed as a conviction that whomever she interacted with would control her. This she experienced in work, at school, in marriage, and in therapy. Continuous efforts were made to relate these "psycho-sick" episodes to what really was going on. Claire gradually recognized that much could be traced to her relationship with her mother, who had dominated her in a seductive and inconsistent way and whose violent words she had tried to hide from. As treatment progressed she became more alert to her feelings as they occurred. After one treatment session that she felt had been "bad" because she had not expressed how she really felt, she closed herself off completely, not only crawling into her cubby hole and closing it off with cardboard, but double-locking all doors. Her feeling was, "My head could have exploded and then it would go into pieces." Instead of dissociating as she had in the past in similar situations, Claire began to think about what might be bothering her, and made a list of the problems that were too much for her. She came up with, and in this order, the therapist, the lab situation, and what might be wrong with herself. This was the beginning of her looking at such episodes as they related to life events, and at the feelings and emotional reactions which she had never clearly recognized. Gradually she understood that she could not define herself by getting into small spaces and that her sense of autonomy needed to be experienced from within, not imposed by external boundaries.

ART WORK

A patient can express himself in many other forms. The exploration of art work is rewarding and revealing, particularly for reconstructing the atmosphere and feeling tone of childhood experiences which many find it difficult to put into words. There is at present a regrettable tendency to subdivide therapy into little subspecialties, with "art therapy" as something separate. It is more useful to include discussion of art work in the general therapeutic investigation. In work with children, play therapy, the use of toys or drawings, is taken for granted in facilitating the expression of conflicts and feelings.

Angela, the young woman mentioned in Chapter Three whose father continuously interfered, had naively asked at first, "Will you teach me how to make decisions?" She was reluctant to believe that her inability to think for herself might be related to what she had experienced as a child. Something like a breakthrough seemed to occur in a session when a childhood anecdote, which she had mentioned rather casually a few days earlier, was analyzed as indicating the basic tragedy of her life, namely that she had felt she was a disappointment to her father. When she was quite young, he had been overseas with the army (World War II) and received photographs of his little girl, who seemed to have blonde curly hair; when he met her at age three she had dark straight hair. Nothing was ever said about his reaction, but the story was told so often, though in a joking way, that Angela became convinced that she was a disappointment to her father and unworthy of his love. She tried to be the super-perfect daughter and her whole life was devoted to fulfilling her father's expectations. She learned early to control her feelings and to display only behavior that was approved by him. As the details of her past life were revealed, she became somewhat more alert to her feeling in relation to different people on the ward; until then she had responded to all with dead-pan disdain or pseudo-friendliness.

At about this time Angela took up a suggestion that had been made at the time of admission, to express her feelings through art work. She took up a device she had enjoyed as a child, applying several layers of crayon and then using a nail to make a design by uncovering the underlying colors. Now it meant to her that the vivid colors expressing violent emotions were hidden underneath the dark controlled surface color, and that by exposing them she could recognize her feelings. By using different pressures in outlining the figures, she indicated the strength of the person and, through various colors, the state of their inner emotions and readiness for emotional rapport.

The leading theme of the series of drawings were the changes in family relationships. The father appeared large, with weak outlines and confused emotions (colors) on the inside. He leaned heavily on the mother, who was represented as a strong figure with more definite emotions, and on his daughter, the patient. In one drawing Angela herself appeared trapped on a dark and narrow road, "pursuing perfection." Gradually she represented herself with changing emotional awareness. In one picture she drew her former self, full of big emotions contained within a strong outline and weak emotions in relation to the environment. On the other half of the same picture, the wall against the world was less sharply defined; the colors indicating inner emotions were less confused, better organized, and able to penetrate the wall. On the day of this drawing the ward psychiatrist remarked that he had for the first time felt in rapport with her, that she had responded with feeling. In the last drawing of this series, she represented herself as taking a new and different road. In a previous picture she stood undecided at a corner. Now she had turned to an open road that permitted an independent development with definable and obtainable goals, and which she called the road of hope. Angela had abandoned the dark, clifflike road which she once pursued in her efforts for perfection and which had no end.

Feeling that she had finished what she had intended to express through her drawings, Angela wanted to take up some other work in occupational therapy. She reported with a certain amusement that the worker asked her, "Aren't you supposed to continue to do your drawings for your doctor?" to which she answered, "My doctor does not tell me what to do. He encourages me to do what I want to do."

As she reconstructed in her art work her concepts of the relationship to her parents, Angela began to take a more active stand against their interference. She finally wrote to them and explained that she was making good progress but that a visit with them at this time would not be helpful, that it might even interrupt what was going on. The father did not reply to her directly but wrote to the therapist instead. In reading this letter she became genuinely angry and indignant about one sentence in which her father demanded a "complete cure" and her becoming "perfectly normal." To her these words contained the kernel of her whole abnormal development, that nothing but the best was good enough for *his* daughter. She also expressed genuine anger and hurt for not having received a direct answer to her letter.

At this time Angela also reported a clearly remembered dream: her dog had died and she cried very much. This meant to her that she was now more in touch with her emotions and more free to express them. This much-loved dog had died when she was fifteen years old, but she had not cried then or had not cried enough. This was further evidence that she had never been allowed to express her true feelings. Angela now explained that her nagging and persistent demand to go home so shortly after admission coincided with her first awareness of genuine feeling, and that she had been afraid to go on with treatment because more feelings might come up.

SCHIZOPHRENIC COMMUNICATION

Attention to the manifold ways of communication is of particular importance in psychotherapy with schizophrenics. Meaningful interpersonal communication is a prerequisite for effective therapy, with understanding and recognition of the implied significance of what a patient says or does not say. Nothing will be accomplished unless the psychiatrist can see meaning in a patient's distorted verbalization, bizarre behavior, and fluctuating attitudes, and in turn conveys this to him. In old-style psychiatry, incoherent communications were conceived of as the random production of a sick mind, presumably stemming from some organic brain disturbance. It was a revolutionary change in psychiatric thinking when it was recognized that schizophrenic illness, whatever its hereditary component, develops under the influence of disturbed interpersonal experiences, which result in aberrant symbolic processes with distortions in perception, meaning, and logic. "Schizophrenese" represents communication on a different level of abstraction, usually more concrete than ordinary language, often rich in puns, unusual analogies, and unlabeled metaphors. During recovery, as a patient learns to function more independently, with more realistic awareness of his own self and a greater capacity for enjoyment of life, the speech patterns also return to normal.

Open-minded readiness and a desire to understand will help in deciphering the often poignant messages. To do this, the therapist needs to draw on his general knowledge and the whole range of his experiences. To illustrate that meaningful communication with a schizophrenic is possible for a beginner, I should like to report an experience from my residency. It concerns Paul, a young man of twenty who was admitted to the clinic for psychotherapy. His illness had started during the previous year when he was working on a defense job (the time was World War II), which involved courses in engineering and mathematics. He had become depressed, could not concentrate, and spoke of his fear of losing his mind—"the calculus is making me sick." He first stayed at a local hospital where he fought against electric shock therapy, which was continued, over a four-month period, in spite of his becoming more agitated and confused; finally he refused to eat, needed tube feeding, and became mute.

When first seen Paul was quiet (under sedation) but he seemed to listen when I spoke to him, reassuring him that at this hospital we were concerned with his problems of living and not with inducing fits in order to make him snap to. He answered slowly and with long pauses between his comments—repeating "That's the idea" and adding that the question was whether to have an old-fashioned house, a wife, and two sons (he was the younger of two brothers) or to live in an apartment with modern equipment and have a son and a daughter. This he repeated several times. He relaxed when it was suggested that as a modern young man he had the right to live a life different from that of his parents and could choose a modern apartment. He brightened up: "That's the idea, a healthy and friendly family."

Paul remained mute most of the time, standing nude in his room, explaining that he was trying to "kill the past in order to step into the present." Clothing was refused because it belonged to the old life, and he gave the same explanation for his refusal to eat, that taking food would only be nourishing the past. He also had to stand up in order to show that he could stand on his own feet. On other days he tried to achieve his goal of "killing the past" by putting his index fingers into his ears, his thumbs against his throat, and the second and third fingers against his nostrils. He kept his mouth tightly closed and was desperate about having to take a deep breath after a while. By that time, enough was known about his background to tell him that he could not undo the past by suffocating himself, or by closing his ears against the constant yelling and nagging of his mother, or by taking her breath away so that she could no longer influence his life.

Concern about his family, and how he could become independent and achieve his own individuality, was the common theme of Paul's various utterances and symbolic acts. At times he was combative and was restrained through wet packs. A new line of comment started with the word "pack," but he used it in terms of a pack of cards. His mother was referred to as the "Queen of Spades, what she says goes." The father was mentioned as the "Deuce, the lowest in the pack." His older brother, whom he admired for having had the courage to emancipate himself, was the "Jack, but in a weaker suit than mother." His own role changed continuously. As the Jack in the same suit as the Queen of Spades he was the closest to his mother but under her continuous domination. He struggled in this delusional game to get away from her, to get an identity of his own; as the King he would be equal to the Queen; as an Ace he would be more powerful but this was dangerous; the Queen might turn the Ace into a One, which "would make him even weaker than the Deuce."

The responses to these various productions were presented in realistic terms. For example, when Paul spoke of his father as the Deuce I commented that it would be hard for the son of such an unimportant person to grow up with a sense of pride; every son wanted to be proud of his father. To this he replied: "And a father wants to be proud of his son," and then went on to talk about his mother in realistic terms. "She lets me use my mind, but only in little ways. I *had* to practice the piano, she yelled and yelled until I did it; but then I could use *my* mind and pick out the pieces I wanted to play."

When he began to speak freely about his background, it was recognized that the real-life interactions within his family had been amazingly similar to what he had expressed during his disturbed period. The mother had been bedridden with arthritis for the past eleven years, dominating the household with her screaming and making them all feel guilty for her suffering. The father was worn out by the tension and sickness in his home. The older brother had always been the leader of the two boys and had managed to liberate himself to some extent. Paul had considered him the only person with whom he could share his feelings but, when he was in turmoil over his own career just before the breakdown, the brother left for the army.

Exactly one month after admission, while talking in his usual schizophrenic manner, he suddenly interrupted himself and said: "I've told enough bull stories. Tell me the honest truth: do people who are as sick as I get well? . . . I've done so much scheming . . . I'm tired of thinking of any more schemes. I want to get well and return to the world." This was not the end of his talking in startling metaphors, but it was his first realistically expressed desire for getting well.

Before the use of psychotropic drugs, patients might communicate in such a style for some time and relapse into it whenever problems appeared overwhelming. Now that the use of tranquilizers shortens the period of psychotic reaction, there is danger that cryptic messages are not listened to. It is essential that the therapist be familiar with the psychotic utterances of his patients because they may contain important information and valuable clues to underlying difficulties. It is much more tedious and time-consuming, and at times impossible, to gain deeper understanding of the problems when these dramatic expressions are completely repressed, or when a patient is not permitted to let it be known how sick he is and to speak about what really troubles him, which he can do during the acute illness only in this indirect way.

Patients seem to be quite aware of the significance of their repetitious, seemingly senseless, utterances. Alice, a young woman from a professional, Protestant background and a gifted musician, had become psychotic shortly before finishing her studies. When admitted to the hospital she was slow-moving, nearly mute but mumbling to herself about the Pope, the Russians, and police horses. With the aid of drugs she lost her psychotic symptoms but was completely apathetic. She was a puzzle to her therapist and to the ward personnel, and there was little or no significant rapport with anyone.

When another therapist took over and showed an outgoing interest in her, Alice gradually opened up and went back to the old preoccupations which had been ignored. During her illness she had avoided all contact with music. As her confidence increased, she began again to listen to records. When she experienced some pleasure at the idea of playing her instrument again, she recalled the painful but urgent concerns experienced during her acute psychosis. She had longed for a "pen pal" behind the Iron Curtain; only somebody enslaved like herself could understand and sympathize with her plight. Though gifted, she had always felt that a musical career had been forced upon her. She had been the youthful member of a family quartet and felt trapped in this role because it was what the family expected. Her hope for salvation was that Pope John would establish a "benevolent dictatorship over the whole world," replacing her parents' implacable demands and ambitions. She had felt a terrific urge to hit a police horse on the rump, thus turning it into a "wild" horse who would then enjoy being alive by running free. With continuous psychotherapy Alice learned that her concept of freedom as running wild was unrealistic. Liberation for her came to mean competence in what she was doing so that she could use her considerable talents for her *own* fulfillment and not as the exploited showpiece of her parents.

In working with such material it is important not to get lost in the symbolic fantasies, but to use them to help a patient obtain a new and clearer understanding of the confusing reality of his life. Such efforts to see meaning in his cryptic and contradictory messages convey to a schizophrenic that what he says is important and maybe even understood. This experience often represents the first step away from the hateful mistrust that separates him from his fellow men. Patients who appear well-oriented and coherent will continue to communicate in the schizophrenic mode or relapse into it when they feel threatened in their tenuous security operations or are confronted again with still unsolved conflicts. It is the therapist's task to recognize the tangible problems that need to be faced without getting sidetracked in the symbolic meaning of the bizarre utterances.

In conclusion I should like again to quote a passage from *I Never Promised You a Rose Garden,* this time to show how a therapist can respond in a meaningful way to schizophrenic shorthand.

"Tomorrow at the same time," the doctor told the nurse and the patient.

"She can't understand you," Deborah said. "Charon spoke in Greek."

Dr. Fried laughed a little and then her face turned grave. "Someday I hope to help you see this world as other than a Stygian hell." (p. 27)

5

On Talking and Listening

The therapist's contribution to therapeutic communication is his ability to listen to what the patient says and conveys through his words and demeanor—and what he leaves out and does not express. This therapeutic listening is not something passive but involves alert and sympathetic participation in what troubles the patient. The therapist must in some measure make "understandable" what the patient experiences in his confused way. This he does through his comments, questions, and responses. His expertise and usefulness lie not in displaying his knowledge of psychodynamics, or what have you, but in his ability to be truly tuned in to a patient and thus help him to discover the roots of his anguish.

To do so he must pay minute attention to what the patient says, including discrepancies in his recall of the past, in the way he misperceives what is happening between him and others, or in how he reacts to the behavior of others or to current events. In particular the therapist needs to be alert to minor manifestations of anxiety, such as hesitation, lowering of voice, disclaiming gestures, changing of subject, or silence. Whatever the symptoms, detailed examination of the circumstances under which they take place, what triggered them off or when exactly they started, usually leads to a more significant understanding of a

patient's problems than immediate focus on this or that unconscious symbolic meaning. It is the therapist's job to hold a
patient to a detailed examination of the when, where, how, and
who in relation to a particular anxiety or disability.

THE BEGINNER'S DILEMMA

Beginners are often anxiously preoccupied with giving insight
to a patient through correct "interpretations." I have been
impressed with how freely they use this particular term. Asking a
question, clarifying an event, defining a feeling tone—everything
is reported as "I gave him an interpretation." He will approach
his first patients with a mixture of feelings: with eagerness
finally to be doing what makes psychiatry the medical specialty
that deals with the psyche, the inner life of people, and with
apprehension that he will be unable to understand his patients or
how to be of use to them in their search for constructive changes
in outlook and functioning. Not uncommonly he harbors the
notion that he should have some specific knowledge and understanding of what underlies a patient's problems and verbal productions.

Student therapists differ considerably in their life experiences
and personalities, in self-confidence, intelligence, integrity, and
objectivity, and in factual knowledge and abilities. All these
factors play a role in the way they will conduct themselves as
therapists. In certain respects doing therapy is more akin to
creative and artistic activity than to definite scientific "technique," a commonly used and unfortunate term. Psychotherapy
is a personal search for understanding, which is not the same for
each therapist or for each patient. It is a sobering discovery to
find out that there is no one "curative insight" or "interpretation" that, if correctly applied, would resolve a patient's problems. The therapeutic encounter is like an initiation. By becoming

intimately acquainted with the inner problems of his patients, the significance of their difficulties, the therapist also becomes aware, in a new way, of his own psychological reactions, his resources of warmth and compassion but also his uncertainties, prejudices, and blind spots. Becoming a psychotherapist is intricately interwoven with developing a professional identity and represents, at the same time, a broadening in one's individuality and maturation as a person.

Being part of a training program in itself creates certain problems. Psychotherapy is essentially a private affair, but during the training period much of what goes on is under the constant scrutiny of others. Students differ in their ambition and need for prestige and recognition, and competition plays an important role. To the extent that this stimulates broader study and greater devotion to work, it is helpful and constructive. But there is the danger that a young therapist will press a patient too hard to produce certain material and information, not guided by the patient's need but by his own desire to give a brilliant psychodynamic discussion in a case conference or to withdraw from a patient who "lets him down" in the eyes of his peers.

THEORETICAL CONCEPTS

The therapist's style of communication reflects his theoretical concepts of personality development and of the aberration reflected in the patient's illness. The therapist who sees his role as that of participant-observer will feel that a patient needs help in facing the painful and confusing realities of his life in order to discover his potentiality for autonomy and self-initiated behavior, in whatever small area this may be possible. He will investigate in collaboration with the patient the vicissitudes of his early development, the times when he experienced anxiety and thus interpreted the world and events around him in a distorted way.

If on the other hand the therapist is convinced that some definite "unconscious" conflict underlies a patient's symptoms, and that this is related to an early trauma or fixation, then he will be preoccupied with uncovering, or guessing, what it was in the hope of giving a good interpretation. In this model the patient is relegated to a more passive role, on the receiving end of the therapist's ministrations.

My expressed concern over a beginner's preoccupation with psychiatric terminology is related to the fact that it might interfere with his therapeutic effectiveness. Learning specific theories and therapeutic techniques, psychoanalytic or otherwise, may be stimulating and give the reassurance that one has been let in on some secret knowledge; to some it may be of help in organizing observations. But the beginner needs to realize that this knowledge does not give him any help when he sits down with a patient. It does not tell you what to say to a patient or what to listen for, and it may even make you focus on something which, according to the theory, should be there and thus stand in the way of hearing what the patient is trying to say.

Many begin with the conviction that to talk along the line of what they actually observe is unprofessional, that it needs immediate translation into the jargon. Instead of thinking in terms of what troubles the patient and how to get along with him in a helpful way, they will be concerned about "defense mechanisms" or "psychodynamics," or become hesitant when unable to make such identifications. On the surface it may not seem to matter whether one refers to Mr. X as doing or saying this or that, or whether one speaks of his having strong or weak ego functions. The telling difference is that in one image the patient is conceived of as a person who is living his own life, though inefficiently and beset with all kinds of problems; in the other, the person is conceived of as a container that houses the various "mechanisms" or "ego functions" which determine what he does.

Premature formulations may stand in the way of learning the truly relevant facts. A therapist who assumes that he already understands the psychodynamics of a patient's problems is not quite so alert and curious in unraveling the unclear and confused periods. He may be tempted to superimpose his preconceived notions on the patient who, because of his sense of helplessness or in order to please the therapist or to reassure himself that treatment is doing him some good, may be only too eager to agree.

Mature therapists have recognized for some time that a patient can achieve self-esteem only by experiencing that what he has to contribute has value, and therefore it is important to let a patient uncover the meaning of his own communication, with the therapist acting as an assistant in the process. If possible a patient should discover this meaning first. The therapist has the privilege to agree or disagree with his conclusions, which makes it important that he be honest and examine the new insight within the total context of the treatment situation and of what he knows about the patient in general. Yet the outmoded model of therapy as interpretation by therapist for patient persists to plague the beginner. The therapist who is too far ahead of his patient in interpreting the meaning of what he has just said may unwittingly repeat one of the most damaging experiences in a patient's background—that "mother always knew what I felt," with the implication that the patient himself did not know what he thought or felt. This style of therapy also reinforces a patient's secret hope that there is some sure-fire answer to his problems and that it will be given to him as a reward for compliant behavior. Clarification of what the patient is saying is best carried out in a manner that enables him to follow it step by step, rather than through disclosure of what to him must seem like some magical incantation; calling it "interpretation" does not change this hidden implication. Much of what the patient says is outside his awareness, "unconscious" to use the common term, but becoming aware of these unknown feelings, fantasies, and attitudes is an active process in which he must participate; otherwise the revelation may reduce him to even greater passivity and helplessness.

More than once I have wondered and worried why young therapists with a seemingly good grasp of a patient's problems, and who seemed to be reporting truthfully and in detail what went on in the treatment sessions, nevertheless were ineffective in their efforts. In one such situation the summarizing statement, when a change of therapist was decided on, clarified the underlying problem: "It seems that Mr. X, although he has superior intelligence and good motivation for therapy, has not been given sufficient insight to immunize him against further attacks of his illness." When I asked the student whether he had really meant to say, "Mr. X has not gained sufficient understanding of his underlying conflicts to be able to handle future difficulties in living without neurotic disturbances," he failed to recognize that there was a difference between the two formulations. This therapist's tendency to superimpose himself upon his patient had been recognized before, and yet the extent to which he had treated him as a passive object on whom he was performing a psychological operation became apparent only in his summary, the verbalization of his basic concept of therapy.

Usually the therapist's concept of the patient as active or passive is expressed in a more subtle way. One young analyst had shown great skill in the treatment of an obsessive young man who felt defeated in his professional aspirations because of a learning block. After the various factors contributing to this inhibition had been brought into the open, the patient finally spoke in realistic terms about taking advanced courses. When the therapist agreed that he was ready for this step, the patient failed to respond with satisfaction and became mildly depressed:

"I think I must stop treatment first. You stand in my way." When this episode was discussed in supervision, the therapist was asked what exactly he had said. It was, "I'll back you up." It could be recognized that the patient's reaction was related to these words which were like the way his mother might express herself. When the question of further schooling came up again, the therapist said simply that the patient could use his sessions to explore all the problems, fears, and fantasies that might come up in connection with the step. Some additional light was thrown on his conflicting feelings about "learning" when the patient recalled with marked affect how his mother had always "translated," from English into English, for his father when they were listening to the radio, repeating word for word what the commentator said, asking impatiently, "You hear? You hear?" The patient had heard something similar, and experienced it as belittling, in the therapist's encouraging remarks. Without direct interpretation and through a difference in wording, the therapist could convey effectively that he, in contrast to the mother, respected the patient's abilities.

To be of help to a patient in gaining useful self-understanding and in becoming more competent and independent, the therapist needs to have a more modest concept of his position and role. The closer a patient and his problems belong to the schizophrenic end of the spectrum of psychiatric disorders, the more likely he is to suffer in his basic self-concept from a profound sense of helplessness, from the fear of being manipulated by outside forces. The therapist's function is to help such a patient uncover and develop his untapped abilities and resources. Neurotics who seemingly function well, except in the area of their unresolved conflicts, often experience doubt about their effectiveness and they, too, will respond positively to a therapeutic approach that encourages self-discovery as an active process.

Filling this more modest role makes definite demands on the

therapist, who must have an open-minded faculty to listen, must be realistic in his self-awareness, must not harbor doubts about his own intellectual ability and professional competence, and must not be competitive with his patients. He must be able to suspend his presumed knowledge so that he can permit a patient to express what he feels and experiences, without having the urge immediately to explain or label what has been said. Neither the patient nor the therapist needs to know the "meaning" of certain statements or behavior, but each must feel free to raise questions and to do it in a way that leads to further clarification. The "meaning" eventually will become apparent.

THE THERAPIST'S STYLE

Communication in psychotherapy is of course a two-way process, but little attention has been paid to the therapist's style of communication. Emphasis throughout the training program is so much on the psychopathology of the patient, and on how to understand his disturbed messages, that when there is failure in understanding it is attributed to the patient's "resistance," misperceptions, or other deficiencies. The possibility that the therapist was unclear or too complex or too learned, or just wrong, is only rarely considered. If the uncovering of unconscious material, or the understanding of complex life situations, is to be therapeutically effective, the way and manner in which this is done is of the greatest importance.

I shall comment here only on some of the more common difficulties beginners are apt to encounter. There is the basic problem of how to talk with a patient, and it is amazing how much this aspect has been neglected in the literature. If self-understanding is a precondition of curative change, the achievement of this understanding is to a large extent dependent on the therapist's ability to establish a process of communication with the patient. It is important that the therapist express indirectly, "I am interested in what troubles you," or "I can see alternatives to your behavior," or "I recognize abilities of which you are not aware." Saying these things in so many words would sound hollow and unfounded, but they can be expressed through the therapist's attitude and his way of listening, questioning, and responding, as well as his nonverbal communication. What he says must convey, in its very texture and tone, respect for the patient, that however confused or distressed he appears now, the therapist respects his basic abilities and his capacity to develop them.

A therapist must be unambiguous and clear in whatever he says, not only to avoid misunderstandings or professional jargon but also to convey that he is open, honest, and warm in his personal interest, and that he has sincere respect for a human being who is struggling to recognize something of value and significance within himself. One needs to establish with each patient a personal style of communication, which without condescension should be geared to the patient's idiomatic ways of expressing himself. Patients respond well to such an open-ended objective attitude focused on finding out what the facts are; they begin to feel that the therapist regards them as collaborators in the search for the unknown factors, and also that the therapist does not have some special knowledge that he is holding back. From consultations on difficult cases, or during the therapy of patients who were previously in treatment, one readily learns that it is not uncommon for a patient to feel that a therapist is withholding knowledge. Conversely, many patients complain that they never understood what they were expected to be talking about, or that they went along with the topics the therapist emphasized even though they meant nothing to them.

At times it is helpful to be explicit about one's attitude and motivation. In the case of a middle-aged professional woman, who was highly indignant about having been sent to a psychiatric hospital on court order after a series of bizarre offenses, a practical situation helped her to recognize that psychotherapy was not just a silly invasion of privacy. "I'd rather go to jail!" had been an often-repeated brushoff. Her driver's license had been suspended and she insisted on going to court to ask for its return. She was furious, even more insulting than usual, when permission was not granted. She responded with startled amazement to her therapist's explanation that she needed to be shielded from further humiliation, that at this moment, with her explosive irritability, no judge would return her license. For the first time she believed at least in the possibility that not all events were specifically designed to inflict new pain and insult on her, and that her physician's attitude contained an element of reliability and trustworthy benevolence.

Most, if not all, of a young therapist's professional communication is with people his equal or superior in rank and prestige, and his way of talking is attuned to this. In the encounter with patients he is dealing with people who, however intelligent and accomplished in certain areas, basically suffer from some deficit in self-esteem and from a readiness to feel they are not valued and respected by others. It is therefore important to formulate what one has to say, and the questions one needs to ask, in a way that does not humiliate a patient by implying his lack of knowledge or understanding, by putting him on the spot, or by making him feel more confused. Among my own teachers it was Sullivan who stressed in his seminars and individual supervision the use of language in this careful way, so that it would give credit to a patient's abilities to understand and express himself, and would avoid making the therapist appear omniscient or above misunderstanding. He specifically warned against such direct questions as "Do you understand me?" when one summarized something, or "What do you mean?" when the patient sounded unclear or contradictory. Instead some indirect comment should be made to clear things up that will not make the patient feel stupid. My own students generally feel that this concern with the formal aspects of what they are saying to their patients is a novel and useful approach. In order to help a patient come to a more objective and realistic understanding of his problems, the young therapist must become sensitive to the quality of his own speech. By acquiring the tools of clear and unambiguous communication he will become more perceptive of what goes on in the therapeutic encounter.

In spite of the wide range of mental disorders, disturbed communication seems to have played a role in most. It is safe to assume that in some respect communication in the family has been unclear, and frequently language was used as much to conceal as to communicate. Sometimes there was endless background chatter without any clear definition of what it was about. At the same time, important issues were not talked about or were directly avoided; they were referred to only by implication, tone of voice, or telling silence. The closer we come to schizophrenic development, the greater the evidence that the style of communication was contradictory, confusing, and inconclusive. If one wants to speak of one basic common error leading to emotional and mental illness, then it is the sin of hypocrisy, of saying one thing and meaning another. Much has been said about the therapist's being effective by the very fact that he responds differently from the people with whom the patient grew up. One important way in which a patient can experience this difference is through the use of language; it should be consistently appropriate, to the point, uncritical and unaccusing. It is not enough for a therapist to claim, "But I am not your mother," when he recognizes signs of inappropriate responses; he must truly behave and talk differently. The honest and predictable use of language is one way in which he can knowingly let a patient experience this difference, without ever spelling it out. In this process of becoming more definite and unambiguous a supervisor can be of direct help to the student therapist.

The therapeutic use of language begins with gathering information about the patient's difficulties and background. This history taking should not be conducted as an inquiry or inquisition, an aggressive questioning about unrelated facts, or an insensitive probing into intimate details. Tact and consideration are particularly needed in exploring sexual development and activities, even in our liberated age and even with patients who flaunt their sexual freedom. Young therapists are apt to feel that they must be free in this area, and some act and talk more freely than they actually feel. Thus they might not be fully alert to a patient's embarrassment, or as tactful in their inquiry and responses as the patient's sensitivities demand.

Since history taking is also part of the therapeutic process, it should be conducted as a supportive common exploration of what the trouble might be. One should avoid questions that can be answered by "yes" or "no"; after that the flow of communication often stops. Even inquiry about as simple a fact as a date should be handled, particularly with an anxious or vague patient, in the form of some suggestion or alternative, such as "Was it before or after summer vacation?" or "Before or after Christmas?" Most of all, the direct question "Why?" should be avoided. For many people it has the background connotation of accusation, or of being declared guilty before the evidence is in. It also carries the implication that there might be a simple concrete answer for what usually is a rather complex and difficult situation with many different determinants. A musing comment along the line of "I wonder what might have played a role in all of this" or "How have you tried to explain it" might start the patient thinking, and when he recognizes the therapist's openminded interest in him, he may even begin to reveal things he has so far held back. Supervision can help a beginner to reformulate comments and questions in a way that is attuned to a patient's needs and problems. Usually this amounts to a simplification of what the student had expressed in a complex or too definite and all-knowing style.

This attention to one's verbal expressions should not result in stilted communication. The important point is that the therapist should learn to recognize that talking with a patient, in particular probing for information, differs from an examination or test situation in the way that questions and answers are related. As he becomes more skillful in his style of inquiry he conveys, in this indirect way, that he is on the patient's side, and thus he activates a potentiality for change that has remained blocked or undeveloped. In this process the therapist develops a precise style of speaking that still reflects his own natural way of expressing himself. It is for this reason that I have kept examples of direct verbal exchanges to a minimum. Each therapist needs to develop his own way of being unambiguous.

EXPLORING FEELINGS

Care in wording one's comments is particularly indicated with a patient who may have been raised with definite inhibitions against expressing spontaneous feelings. Others may be embarrassed about having "vulgar" emotions, or may have trained themselves not even to acknowledge them. Patients need help in identifying and expressing their feelings, but this must be done in a way that it is not shocking or insulting. A sure showstopper is, "You must have been very angry, or jealous . . ." If it brings a confirming response, the patient may feel either that he has been found out or that the doctor is a mindreader. It is usually more productive to offer a question that indicates the area in which one expects information, but the question should be given as an alternative. When confronted with a patient who is particularly reluctant to talk about his family, or whose whole history and demeanor indicate that he never has expressed his feelings, one might ask, "Who in your family was permitted to show his temper, or did they all practice a stiff upper lip?" If "stiff upper lip" is chosen as the answer, then one has the opening of inquiring how this was conveyed as a desirable stance, whether by rigid example or outspoken admonition, and how the rule was broken.

A reproachful insistence that the patient is resisting or not telling what he really feels may only provoke resentment or a temper outburst when the patient feels pushed too far—it rarely leads to meaningful exploration of the underlying issues. I recall Ida, a girl of eighteen, of whom the resident reported that she was negativistic and refused to talk about her family, always repeating that nothing was the matter with them. In an interview with me, in the presence of the resident, she was equally reluctant, stating repeatedly that "nothing ever happened." I took this phrase as my cue and confirmed, "Then you had a childhood of nonhappenings." My use of the colloquialism made her smile and she opened up. Actually her statement had been quite correct: Ida's childhood had not been characterized by any describable traumatic events, but she had suffered from true deprivation in emotional responses and personal support. Many of the positive confirming experiences that a child needs for confident and competent development had simply never taken place. She was a late-born child who came along when her older siblings were already troublesome teenagers. The only message she had clearly heard during her childhood was that it would have been better had she not been around.

People who have grown up under such emotionally deprived circumstances may be truly lacking in the ability to identify feeling tones. Thus they are not just denying or avoiding something when they say that they do not feel anything or do not know how they feel. With such patients a beginner may experience difficulties in recognizing implied feeling tones, and he needs help in recognizing the minor manifestations of uneasiness and discomfort which may point to unidentifiable feelings. He needs to learn how to assist a patient in developing awareness of the appropriate feeling response to some painful or exciting experience. Otherwise he is in danger of becoming impatient or disappointed when a patient does not respond to what he has so carefully pointed out as the trouble. The difficulty may not lie in the correctness or incorrectness of the deduction but in the vocabulary used for describing emotional states. It is easy to recognize that complex concepts need clarifying, but it is much more difficult to discover that everyday terms may be without real meaning to a patient who has never had the chance to organize his concepts or vocabulary along these lines.

Some time ago I saw in consultation Nora, a young woman who had made little progress during several years of psychiatric treatment. She was impressive in her exaggerated use of expletives and crude remarks, through which she tried to demonstrate that therapy had "liberated" her. While reviewing her life history she mentioned that her first awareness of being "different" was when she had felt nothing at the death of a grandfather to whom she had been closely attached. Nora had gone through life mimicking what she saw her contemporaries express as feelings, but she was quite aware there was no real substance below her surface behavior. Her former therapist recognized correctly that she had never been encouraged to express her anger and what looked like suppressed rages, but he did not see that these terms had no meaning for her. She needed help to learn carefully to recognize and differentiate her own feeling responses in a variety of situations.

A similar problem was encountered in Nathan, a thirteen-year-old Jewish boy who showed rapid changes in behavior following his bar mitzvah. Until then he had been the bright hope of his family. He became preoccupied with guilt, feeling an urgent need for atonement of his sins. This overshadowed his thinking and he developed a whole series of rituals; he explained whatever he did or did not do as being motivated by fear of guilt. No progress was made in therapy until attention was paid to the broad area of feeling tones which he never mentioned and which he said, when asked, he did not experience. Nathan had grown up in a family in which "not giving trouble" and "taking it" were praised as virtues. It was gradually worked out that the sensation he called "guilt" was aroused whenever there was the slightest manifestation of any other feeling in him and for which the appropriate term might have been "anger," "anxiety," "bodily discomfort," or "demands" based on them. It took great patience on the part of the therapist to pursue these manifestations of tension and discomfort, and to help the boy recognize their importance in the whole pattern of his development, instead of pursuing, as had been done until then, the possible events that might have aroused so much guilt.

DEFINING THE RELATIONSHIP

Not infrequently, patients and beginning therapists share the popular notion that a patient keeps on talking and talking, something called "free association," and that the psychiatrist will cure him by telling him what it all means. Even the most rigidly orthodox psychoanalyst would consider this description a caricature of the analytic process, though young therapists may attempt to adhere to such a model and an unsuspecting supervisor may not immediately recognize this. It is, of course, in some ways easier to let a patient go on talking instead of clarifying the underlying issues by astute questions. A patient may express in his statements rather distorted views of events and relationships. The listener must be aware that, by not challenging them then and there, he expresses agreement according to the principle that "silence is consent."

In particular there is need to define the therapeutic relationship and to discourage tactfully the development of an overintense attachment. An unsure beginner can misuse the therapeutic relationship to bolster his own security needs. By taking at their face value a patient's admiration or declaration of dependency, and silently accepting it instead of exploring its significance, he will encourage a "positive transference" to a dangerous degree. Severe difficulties may develop when a therapist's need for reassurance interacts with a patient's demands for special recognition, sometimes openly expressed as a demand for love. Acute psychotic episodes may occur under such conditions.

Take the case of Mrs. A, a thirty-year-old woman who had left college to marry at age twenty and then had several children in quick succession. She was disappointed in her husband, who was rather insecure himself and who decided to leave his company in the midwest to look for better opportunities in the east. This move meant for both husband and wife the severing of relationships with their families and old friends. While getting established in the new home, Mrs. A suffered an acute psychotic episode from which she recovered during a brief hospitalization. She was enthusiastic about continuing as a private patient with the same therapist and openly expressed her admiration for him. Things seemed to be going well, so well indeed that after a few months her family felt that the expense for treatment was dispensable. She told her doctor, "I can't afford you any more," and, without going into it further, he agreed to discontinue treatment. She was upset when she left his office, sat in her car until she saw his next patient leave, and then returned to his office, asking him to kiss her. When he refused she advanced toward him and he took her face into his hands, kissed her lightly on the cheek, and said, "You have to go now; I'm going to miss you, old funny face."

At this moment Mrs. A became consciously convinced that their relationship had been really an "affair," that there had always been something special between them. She always had the feeling that she did not need to say anything, that he always "knew" what was on her mind and that they understood each other without words. She had expressed active interest in him as a person, in his family and his private life, something he neither encouraged or discouraged and never openly discussed. She was sure that he "felt" the same way about her as she did about him. Now she became acutely concerned about whether their affair was known, whether people were following her to see if it was continuing; she became obsessed with the idea that something forbidden had gone on and that the "illicit relationship" might harm him, that the medical authorities might be out to get him. She telephoned his office repeatedly and asked him to marry her; he sent her to a pharmacy for tranquilizing drugs. Mrs. A now became obsessed with the feeling that she had been rejected. She tried to commit suicide by taking all the pills in her possession and then attempted to cut her throat with a kitchen knife. Her husband found her in the bathroom and brought her back to the hospital.

This sequence of events was gradually elucidated by Mrs. A's new therapist, also a resident, whom she attempted to involve in a similar tacit "affair." Since he worked under supervision he became alert to and openly discussed her ingratiating and seductive ways. She was contemptuous at his insistence on their having to be open about what was going on between them, and she became quite aggressive. She continued to demand to be understood without words and was indirect in everything she said, always insinuating that there was something erotic in the nature of their relationship. By not accepting her insinuations, and by being honest in defining the nature of the relationship, the new therapist helped her to realize that "love would not cure her," contrary to her continued demands. Only after this did Mrs. A become involved in a meaningful therapeutic relationship, in which her feelings were stated and explored. It is only too understandable that the beginner feels reassured when a patient expresses special appreciation for him and his skill. Usually the consequences of dismissing such an admiring attitude are not quite so dramatic. Yet permitting a dependent "positive transference" to prevail is definitely nontherapeutic.

6

On Teaching and Learning

Psychotherapy is conducted as an encounter between two people, the patient and the therapist, and what is communicated in this intimate relationship is essentially private. Yet in some respects, during the training period, the therapeutic process is only semi-private, when the therapist reports to a supervisor about his experiences with a particular patient; sometimes it is semi-public, when he discusses a patient in a case seminar; and other times it is more or less public, when a patient participates in a case conference and is interviewed in front of an audience. These various violations of the condition of privacy modify what goes on in the individual treatment sessions, but not always in an undesirable way.

GRAND ROUNDS

I have attended more than one case conference where a patient who had been described as reluctant and resistant blossomed out and "told it all," as if having his day in court. Under unfavorable conditions a tactless interviewer, not considering the patient's sensitivities, may open up problems for which neither the patient nor the therapist is prepared. For the student therapist, although these various teaching procedures may provide the help he expects in his efforts to learn, he may experience them as harsh exposure to the criticism of his peers and teachers. At its best, however, the grand-rounds presentation demands from him a review of the patient's development, an organization of the mass of material he has accumulated and how it relates to what has gone on in therapy, and a comparison of his experience with what has been reported in the literature. All this is a positive stimulus toward a maturing self-assessment.

Customarily in such conferences another psychiatrist is invited to discuss the presentation according to his own view of the matter. Few experiences are more stimulating and enriching than following an experienced therapist spell out in detail his thinking on the problems of a patient and the way he applies his deductions to the therapeutic process. Such a discussion can open up new and unexpected vistas. To be of didactic help, such a discussion should be relevant to the student's stage of experience. Unfortunately, I have attended innumerable conferences and case presentations where the discussant expressed only stereotyped clichés of the established theory; he recited advanced points of psychoanalytic theory and metapsychology which were neither relevant to the case under discussion nor of any possible significance to the students. What a student can learn from this, however, is that there are verbal maneuvers which seem learned and informed without making any sense; the hidden message is that they add to one's prestige.

ELECTRONIC TEACHING AIDS

Recordings or videotaped interviews and treatment sessions are increasingly being used for teaching purposes. They have the great advantage of sparing a patient the embarrassment of revealing his innermost thoughts and feelings in front of strangers. They permit discussion of what is going on in detail, and when something is relevant or unclear certain sections can be replayed. These methods help in many ways to increase a beginner's skills, his ability to listen carefully to what the patient says explicitly and to recognize the implicit meanings. He can be taught to become more alert to the nonverbal signals of a patient and, even more important, to his own verbal and nonverbal expressions—how he reinforces a patient in what he communicates and thus encourages him to go on and open up or, conversely, how by forbidding gestures, irrelevant questions, or uncalled-for changes of subject, he may keep the patient from saying what he seemed to be ready to express.

There is great demand for being shown how one actually "does" psychotherapy. More sophisticated students may ask, "What are some of the ways to do it?" It appears to me that, although these various methods are useful for learning *about* psychotherapy, one cannot learn how to do it oneself from watching others. Watching experienced therapists interview patients may show the beginner that each proceeds in a different style, and he thus learns that he too must develop his own assets. Some will find it encouraging that he can develop in a way that is honestly in agreement with his personality and what he feels when listening to a patient. Others are confused by the fact that there are so many individual variations and different styles; they want definite "how to" prescriptions.

Observing therapeutic sessions is more productive when a senior therapist attends, makes running comments, and is available for discussion afterwards. I recall one occasion when I together with a resident group observed a therapeutic session on closed-circuit television. Things seemed to be going well and the patient talked about important issues. It appeared that she had decided ahead of time to bring some special difficult problems into the open. About halfway through the session the therapist began first gently, then more vigorously, to tap one foot—it did not distract the patient, who continued with what she had on her mind.

Finally, toward the end of the session, the therapist brought a particularly important issue to the attention of the patient. I commented, "Oh, that's what the tapping was about," and only one of the residents had also noted it. When the therapist was asked about this afterwards, he realized that he had begun to feel impatient about not getting a chance to say what was on his mind. He had planned to bring the topic up fairly early in the session because he felt the patient should have ample time to react to it, but since she was talking spontaneously about important problems, he had to postpone what he wanted to say. Only the tapping indicated his preoccupation.

However well presented recorded sessions are technically, with their advantage of allowing one to stop at various significant points, they lack the underlying tension and aliveness that is part of every treatment session, the unexpressed and unverbalized possibilities that the therapist, or the patient, consider but discard. Absent is the whole atmosphere of alert attention that keeps you involved when you do not know what is going to happen next. Still, I do not wish to underrate the importance of indirect learning through observation. On the contrary, these various devices are excellent for demonstrating clinical syndromes, and they help to sharpen the beginner's acumen for detailed and systematic observation and description of symptoms and behavior. Group discussions of taped interviews can also demonstrate what is meant by psychodynamic constellations, defense mechanisms, and such, and thus they help the beginner to become more observant and articulate about what is going on with his own patients. Continuous case seminars on the therapeutic treatment of one or two patients, during which the listeners take part in the discussion, are informative in a similar way. However, they cannot take the place of individual supervision.

INDIVIDUAL SUPERVISION

It has been objected that individual supervision is too time-consuming and that group supervision is just as efficient. This is doubtless correct for the more general teaching aspects, but it works less well in terms of the therapist's need to develop an awareness of the subtleties of his personal involvement. During the supervision of advanced students in groups of two or three, I have noted repeatedly that they established a rotating drop-out system, explaining that they preferred to have one-to-one supervision, though less often, because it was more meaningful; they felt they learned relatively little from listening to what the others reported. Sharing the supervision, they thought, prevented them from being quite so open about themselves, less free to ask questions, and less responsive to suggestions.

Though supervision takes up a great deal of time in most teaching programs, very little has been written on it. What has been published deals mainly with the supervision by analysts of psychoanalytic candidates who can no longer be considered beginners. Almost nothing has been written on supervising the raw beginner. Yet it is he who is most in need of this intimate and specialized assistance, and whether his development takes a positive or unfavorable direction may be decisively influenced by his experiences with supervisors. The need for teaching through personal preceptorship is determined by the special problems of the psychiatric residency, which differs in many ways from the residency in other medical specialties. Becoming a psychotherapist is a very personal experience and requires highly individualistic learning.

An important factor is that the preparation in medical school for psychotherapy has been rather deficient. The skills the future therapist acquires during his student years are based more or less on hard-fact observation and action, be it direct operation on the patient (electro-shock therapy in psychiatry), prescription of drugs, or evaluation of environmental stress. In contrast, the tools the psychotherapist needs are his own personality, his sensitivity to interpersonal processes, and his own reactions in the relationship to patients; they are shaped by his own feelings about himself and others. Basically psychotherapy represents a study of the difficulties and distortions encountered with a patient who has been exposed during his development to confusing and hurtful relationships that often were judgmental, rejecting, unbending and dishonest, and which may have left him mistrustful of any new involvement. A major force in bringing about beneficial change through psychotherapy is the very newness of this particular human relationship, which, if effective, encourages greater independence and self-assertion.

Some psychiatric residents are practicing physicians who decide on a new career because they wish to increase their skills in helping patients with various psychological problems. Their greater maturity is an asset, but they may find it difficult to switch to a new concept of doctor-patient interaction, where the doctor's role is more that of a catalyst in encouraging the patient to acquire greater competence. Others find it hard to accept the fact that progress is relatively slow, and they become concerned about not doing the patient any good, that they are wasting his time and money. These psychologically oriented physicians usually have had the experience of patients reacting to them in a grateful and trusting way. It comes as a shock when they discover that during intensive therapy patients, instead of being pleasant, express doubts, are openly hostile, try to control the interview, or attempt to manipulate the therapist.

Beginners vary widely in the problems they experience while developing an evocative therapeutic attitude. But basic to the process is a deepened sense of one's own identity. Of course the beginner expects the supervisor to help him recognize what troubles his patients. Yet he needs just as much, if not more, assistance in developing his own person into an effective therapeutic instrument, and this requires highly individualized teaching.

STYLES OF SUPERVISION

Student therapists are exposed to a great variety of supervisory approaches, ranging from discussion of their patients with a trainee a year or two ahead of them, or with a young faculty member, to supervisory sessions with experienced therapists and analysts. There is variety of approach in the content of what supervisors teach as well as in their method. I am in the habit of asking my students for detailed information about their experiences with other supervisors. There are many differences in the way students are required to proceed: some teachers let them develop their own method of reporting; others want detailed written notes, with attention to the meaning of individual words and statements. Some focus from the beginning on what the patient "feels" about the therapist, others on what the patient reveals about his childhood and past experiences. Some residents experience this diversity as confusing, others as enriching and helpful in becoming familiar with a variety of viewpoints.

Supervisors vary widely in their concepts of what a student needs to learn and how he should be taught. Parallels are drawn between theoretical concepts of the nature of mental illness and concepts of the essence of the therapeutic process. One who conceives of mental illness as an expression of unconscious conflicts, and who considers insight into them as curative, will be more inclined to instruct the student in the underlying psychodynamics. Those who consider the clarification of a patient's difficulties with people as the essence of the therapeutic process, and who feel that his difficulties are related to the inadequate guideposts and often blatant misinterpretations by which he lives, will focus on subtle distortions in communication, with stress on the interactional experiences between patient and therapist.

There is of course no one method of supervision suitable for all. How an individual student should proceed depends on the way his memory functions and the ease with which he can combine note taking and listening. He needs to train his memory and to review each session after the patient has left, writing down the main topics and significant patterns. In particular he should reconstruct the movement from one topic to another, whether he or the patient changed the subject and at what point and for what purpose. Whatever method of note keeping one prefers, it is important for the student to review what has gone on with his patients before each supervisory session and to present this summary first. In my experience few follow these suggestions when they are made, and continue to proceed in the way that suits their current needs; yet with growing feelings of competence and independence, they will develop a style of reporting that usually is quite close to that suggested here. The inability to follow such a broad outline reflects the student's problems with the task itself.

Recorded sessions may be helpful when a beginner has unusual difficulties in perceiving and reporting what has gone on between him and his patient. Reviewing a recorded interview with a supervisor may be helpful in making a student aware of his awkward style of communication or of his lack of attention to subtle but important points. He may have tuned his patient out and then, not having grasped what was said, change the topic. Joint listening to a tape is a useful exercise, but it does not replace a student's learning to take notes appropriately and developing the skill to organize in his mind what has come up in a session. He must gradually learn to discern what is relevant.

Taping an interview cannot possibly duplicate the learning experience of reviewing events in one's mind and reporting this personal summary. In actual work with a patient we have to rely on memory and the associations that come up in context when we put various points together and use them for appropriate responses. Reporting in supervision is good training for learning to trust one's memory. A student who is not able to condense the relevant aspects of a session, and who does not communicate well with his supervisor, usually is also handicapped in carrying out psychotherapy.

Like psychotherapy itself, the supervisory process often begins with considerable misperceptions and defensive maneuvers. This may express itself in the way a resident talks about his different supervisors, which reflects as much about his personality and ways of reacting as about the actual procedures. The same supervisor may be described by one resident as "Difficult—he isn't interested in what I say. He likes to talk about the unconscious and explain what the patient really means," and by another as "Very helpful—he tells me exactly what things mean and what to do." Another supervisor may be described by one student as "Encouraging—he lets me figure things out, and then makes a relevant comment," and by another as "Too vague—I never know what he's after and he doesn't really teach me anything." These abbreviated comments reflect a broad range of supervisory styles but, even more, the range of residents' attitudes and expectations, from the passive dependent expectation of being "instructed" to greater self-reliance or even reluctance to accept anything coming from anybody else. These different approaches to the learning process can also be recognized in varying attitudes toward patients. The supervisory process needs to be geared to the learner's flexibility, reliance on his own judgment, and capacity for genuine involvement.

With all the differences, there seems to be an increasing

emphasis on functional processes rather than on conflicts and traumatic events. Somewhat paradoxically, it appears that the younger teachers are more rigid and tradition-bound; perhaps still too close to the effort invested in their own training, they pass on as facts what they have been taught. Not having had the time and clinical experience to let their special knowledge ripen, they are apt to transmit outdated theoretical concepts, without considering possibilities that the theory does not prescribe. This adherence to old models, which makes psychiatric training so confusing, appears to be related to the traditionalism of the younger generation of teachers. Some are quite directive, even authoritarian, insisting that a student confront or "hit" a patient with whatever they have inferred is the correct interpretation.

One might have assumed the opposite, that the young teachers have the great advantage of being closer to a beginner's problems and that the student therapist would feel more free in expressing doubts and anxieties to them. There are of course young supervisors who are aware of the learner's special problems and encourage him to develop his own style, who look upon his doubts and questions as an asset and not as something to be hidden behind a mask of pseudo-certainty.

INTERACTIONAL PATTERNS

The supervisory experience represents a complex system of communication and interaction. The task is to help the student therapist be effective with a particular patient as he also learns by doing. In this process he needs to become aware of his personal assets and liabilities, and he must learn the principles of psychotherapy so that he can apply them to those patients whose treatment is not supervised. The material in the hands of the supervisor initially may be rather unreliable: he has to depend on what the student reports about his patient, and this may be out of focus. Much of what the student reports reflects his own difficulties and his not always objective perception of the patient's problems. At the same time, his approach to the supervisor may be determined by his own habitual responses to "authority figures" rather than by the personal qualities and demands of the supervisor. Since supervisors differ so widely in their concepts and approach, rather complex patterns of interaction develop. Just as during therapy not every unproductive period of tension is a reflection of a patient's "resistance," so too not every difficulty in supervision indicates an inhibition in the student.

Some residents start doing therapy with a sense of independence; usually they had some past experience when they were on their own and approached their patients with the open attitude of "let's see what we can do together." They may initially experience the structure of residency and supervision as limiting, as interfering with their freedom and spontaneity. They may have difficulties with rigid or inexperienced supervisors who want to superimpose definite theories or to whom teaching means indoctrination. In others the stance of independence may mask a secret conviction of superiority or a fear that, if there is still something they need to learn, they will be revealed as deficient, less than superior. In contrast, others may see the teacher as an omniscient being who will satisfy their needs and impart knowledge without their having to make the effort to participate actively in the learning process. Still others are more preoccupied with impressing the supervisor and may be openly competitive with him.

Clarification of disturbed communication and of interfering emotional attitudes is an important aspect of supervision. As the student becomes more secure and open in his relationship to the teacher, as a certain trusting atmosphere develops, his capacity for more reliable observation increases and his reports become a more valid measure of what the patient is expressing. If reports about what goes on in therapy continue to be foggy, studying a recorded session, or interviewing the patient together with the student, may help to resolve the problems by revealing some of the distortions that have resulted in omission or misrepresentation of important factors.

As a supervisor I prefer to interview a patient when there is an impasse in therapeutic progress. Sometimes a student therapist expresses concern that this might interfere with the transference relationship or undermine the patient's confidence in him. But invariably patients respond with some expression of relief—they had expected that in a teaching hospital the more experienced staff members would stand by as consultants. I do not recall a single incident where such a joint interview interfered with the therapeutic relationship; usually a patient will add the therapist's willingness to learn to the list of his assets.

Some students are so rigidly set in feeling intimidated by a supervisor that no constructive learning takes place; such a student will also be handicapped in relating to his patients. At times, changing to a supervisor with whom the student feels more comfortable may be of help. Usually, however, continuous difficulties reflect the student's own problems and he should be advised to seek therapeutic help for himself. There are also situations where therapist and patient are poorly matched, or where a student is clearly unable to help a patient, and then it is the supervisor's responsibility to suggest a change of therapist for that patient.

In successful individual supervision, a personally meaningful relationship develops that cannot take place in classroom instruction. As understanding and agreement build up about the valid issues to be explored, the student becomes more amenable to suggestions from his supervisor, not as authoritarian instruction but as procedure worked out on the basis of mutual and collaborative understanding. As the student gains in understanding his own reactions to the patient, he becomes more consistent in the way he responds to him, more aware of distortions in the patient's account or of contradictions and omissions. Continued supervision helps him to become increasingly skillful in recognizing deviations in the patient's communication. He is more open in his readiness to learn, less determined to exhibit that he knows it already, less concerned with hiding his ignorance. Thus he becomes more effective in eliciting in his patient the desire to change, the readiness to reexamine past difficulties and relationships in a new way.

DEVELOPING SELF-AWARENESS

As stated earlier, a supervisor's teaching of psychotherapy closely parallels his concept of the therapeutic process. In my view, the treatment process must lead to a patient's improving deficient tools of self-awareness, self-presentation, and communication, and his acquiring the capacity to rely on his own thinking and feeling, becoming more realistic in his self-appraisal and more aware of his patterns of interacting with others. If "insight" is the goal of therapy, it should not be conceived of as something imparted by others but as the kind of self-understanding acquired only by actively working toward the goal. Similarly, I conceive of learning psychotherapy as an active process, which a student achieves through communication and interaction with his supervisors.

In the preceding chapter I discussed the importance of clear speech for therapeutic communication. Attention in supervision to the student's way of talking is vital. To the degree a student is open in verbal exchanges with his supervisor, his communication with patients will improve. Awareness of style of communication fosters confidence in the beginner; confronted with seemingly confused and contradictory situations, he has the inner assurance of "I know how to clarify things." A premature emphasis on "where the patient is going" may leave him worried about having missed some fine points or make him anxious about having made a mistake.

During supervision he receives advice on how to keep the interview going, in particular with patients who are inhibited or depressed or who have led such lonely lives that they cannot be immediately articulate in talking about themselves. By reviewing with his supervisor what he has gathered from the patient's past history as well as the ongoing interaction with him, the young therapist may gain a new perspective on what is going on, and this he can use to show the patient that his problems can be understood in a fresh way. It is just as important for him to become alert to what he himself is doing: the more relaxed, clear, and open-minded he is, the greater the chance that the patient will feel understood. The supervisor can help to clarify what the patient expresses as his real problem, or how to help him deal in a constructive way with what the therapist has observed.

UNSTATED MESSAGES

Not uncommonly, a supervisor will pick up something the student did not report because he was unaware of its possible therapeutic significance. Earlier I drew attention to hidden ways of expressing conflictual material through everyday acts and experiences that are not explicitly mentioned in therapy. An example was the patient who was late because he was embarrassed about inheriting his father's limousine. Similarly, a young therapist may condone certain attitudes in a patient without realizing the message they contain. I wish to give only one example, that of a therapist who was skillful in listening and responding to a patient, a gifted student who had worked her way through college and was now working her way through medical school. In spite of good evidence of unusual competence, she suffered from episodes of depression and feared that she might become too anxious when required to do responsible work on the clinical services. The therapist reported in detail on the background of this unreasonable anxiety and on the direction in which they were going to pursue the problem. In a different context the therapist mentioned in passing that the student was also considering an academic career, so that she did not need to anticipate such anxiety after graduation, and they had discussed several practical possibilities. The resident was rather surprised when it was pointed out that this discussion must have conveyed to the patient a negative message, namely that the therapist also felt she had no chance of liberating herself from these crippling anxiety states and that thereby he was denying the whole purpose of therapy: a patient's achievement of greater self-esteem and confidence.

There are many other unstated problems that require a supervisor's alert attention. Not infrequently the young therapist takes the patient's reports about background experiences, particularly the relationship to the mother, at face value and proceeds as if these anxiety-ridden childhood images are still valid: the mother continues to be experienced as all-powerful and controlling, and is not viewed as the bewildered, even pathetic person she may be. Beginners may go to great lengths to avoid the reproach of "you are just like my mother" and may be more permissive, or "understanding," than is justified. Others may be unaware of the extent to which they superimpose their own values on a patient. Frequently this comes out through expressions of the same expectations as the culture at large, which the patient experiences as "like my parents." If this factor is not clearly recognized, treatment of a seemingly promising patient—and we are apt to put intelligent and articulate young patients in this category—may result in a stalemate, the more so the "better" the performance. A supervisor can help a beginner to recognize how such a promising person must develop the capacity to feel self-directed before he can venture out on his own.

SUPERVISION AS THERAPY

Supervision is intended to enhance a beginner's alertness to what is going on in him and with his patient. This very personal way of instruction does not take the place of individual psychotherapy, though many residents experience it as helpful and some call it "therapeutic." There are several situational similarities, such as meeting regularly for the student's benefit; and as in other interpersonal situations in which one seeks help and one provides help, "transferred" feeling tones and attitudes will appear. When the student can express them openly, or can accept correction when attention is drawn to inappropriate responses, a corrective reevaluation of his patterns of reacting takes place. I am inclined to consider this beneficial effect of supervision in the light of other positive and corrective life experiences. It is different from psychotherapy, where one investigates the factors underlying such behavior.

Supervision provides many opportunities to broaden the therapist's range of self-awareness—it encourages him to be explicit about attitudes that usually remain unexpressed and helps him to recognize competitive and prestige strivings for what they are, not as rationalizations for his behavior with a patient. Many need support in accepting the fact that as learners they are entitled not to know something and to overlook certain points that the supervisor recognizes. If he cannot accept instruction and correction but reacts with undue self-incrimination or sullen anger for having been found wanting, the student may himself need direct therapeutic help (which would involve a type of inquiry that is beyond a supervisor's responsibility).

Moralistic attitudes that may stand in the way of the therapist's effectiveness are also modified during supervision, and it works in both directions. Someone coming from a rigid conventional background may be shocked—something he is apt to conceal—when he learns about the wide range of and frantic search for sexual experiences through which distressed people try to escape their loneliness and personal uncertainty; for him, becoming familiar with the way a life is lived without judging it is a broadening experience. Others who are aggressively liberal in their sexual attitudes need guidance in accepting that not every girl who wants to be a virgin when she marries is a narrow-minded and repressed Victorian prude, and that she deserves respectful support for her decision to adhere to traditional standards. The beginner needs support as he becomes anxious and impatient when progress is not dramatic, and not as rewarding as his own need for reassurance demands; in particular he must be restrained from declaring a patient "untreatable" when he feels he has failed and wants to recommend some organic treatment method instead.

Though ill-defined, certain characteristics of attitude and interpersonal experience seem to be essential for effective work as a psychotherapist. These qualities are usually referred to as maturity and self-awareness, security and self-respect; good supervisory experiences may foster their development. Doing psychotherapy requires the ability to listen to others without letting your personal problems and frustrations, or prejudices and preconceived notions, interfere with being fair, firm, and honest. Some degree of depression, irritability, impatience, helplessness, pessimism, or discouragement is probably experienced by all at one time or another, not only by the beginner. Such reactions need to be recognized lest defensive maneuvers to preserve your own self-esteem render you deaf to the communication and needs of your patients.

7

The Therapeutic Experience

Psychotherapy confronts a patient with the underlying deficits or contradictions in his personality. By clarifying them he acquires new ways of coping with the tasks and demands of living without suffering undue anxieties or reviving old unresolved conflicts, and without needing to escape into invalidism, depression, or uncontrolled impulsiveness. This does not mean that as a result of psychotherapy all the difficulties of living will disappear, though demanding patients may hope for just that and an enthusiastic beginner may feel that he has failed when he does not achieve it. "I Never Promised You a Rose Garden," the cautionary statement of a master therapist, succinctly expresses the limitations of what can reasonably be achieved.

A beginner asks what the elements are of the change to greater competence and courage. Summaries of treatment histories are in some ways misleading because of their focus on highlights and positive findings. Reading about treatment cannot give more than hints of various aspects of the change, the ups and downs in mood and rapport. It cannot be repeated too often: the realities of the process can be learned only by doing therapy.

No definite procedure can be given which would be applicable to all patients or suitable for all therapists. Though patients are most harassed by their immediate problems and symptoms, it is useful, and in the long run essential, to recognize fairly early an underlying central dynamic issue, particularly in complicated cases, those with long histories and repeated changes of symptoms. Pursuit of the one or other symptom may lead to the recognition of interesting symbolic meanings, but it rarely results in the resolution of the illness. It is important to pursue whatever the patient offers; by looking at the problem from various angles and in different perspectives, a central issue will become apparent sooner or later. The amount of information for any one patient is like a tangled mass of many threads and pieces: you have to get hold of one thread and begin to unravel the tangle.

There has been much debate in recent years about the relative importance of the therapeutic investigation of current problems as against investigation of childhood memories. With an open-ended and open-minded attitude there will be continuous oscillation in the focus of attention: an upheaval in the present will be examined in view of a similar crisis in the past; a faulty attitude behind today's conflicts will be traced to distorting childhood experiences; and a patient's reactions to the therapist and his concept of the doctor-patient relationship will be related to experiences with people in his current or past life. To illustrate how problems that arise in the course of treatment offer the material with which to work, I shall give here a few brief sketches of extended treatment histories.

THE CASE OF THE FORMER NUN

Anna, briefly described in Chapter Three, who on first impression appeared so meek and submissive, got things going in therapy by her defiant refusal to be seen by a medical student. To her surprise, this was handled not as a disciplinary problem but as a therapeutic message. She herself focused on two points: she wanted to make sure that the clinic, unlike the convent where she suffered her breakdown, would not coerce her into obedience, and she hoped that her therapist, though inexperienced, would recognize the importance of the step and have the courage to back her up. Both points proved to be of importance to the resolution of Anna's problems. In view of her pride in her many therapeutic failures, it was drawn to her attention—and she accepted it in the semi-joking way in which it was offered—that if she proved to herself that her new doctor had courage, then she would be an even greater and more powerful "invalid" if she succeeded in defeating yet another therapeutic effort.

To avoid any misunderstanding: such a refusal needs to be evaluated in the context of each patient's total situation. Because of Anna's background history and her severe anxiety, lenient acceptance appeared indicated in her case. Other situations require an entirely different approach. One eighteen-year-old boy, with anorexia nervosa of six years' standing, was highly manipulative and lived in constant fear of being taken advantage of. He repeatedly objected to being interviewed by medical students— there was no sense in cooperating, he felt, since he was not gaining any benefit. His fear of being "used" was made the focus of the therapeutic inquiry, and he finally admitted that he learned something from this experience; from then on he took part in interviews with students.

To return to Anna: the role of obedience in her life was explored in its many ramifications, especially as it related to the constant state of anxiety that made her reject any planned routine activity and the mistrust with which she reacted to the staff. An entirely new picture of her early development evolved. During her previous hospital admission she had been described as having no neurotic traits as a child. Family relationships were rated as satisfactory and noncontributory to her illness: "A happy home, with a kindly mother as the center of the household. Patient liked to play with boys and was happy. She had cared for the younger five children and worried about them." All her siblings were stable and had families of their own, and there were no other clerics in her family. During the new evaluation she confessed that she had felt abused in her childhood, that as the oldest girl she was expected to be her mother's untiring helper and to relieve her of the burden of caring for five younger children and an older crippled brother. These demands were made not directly by the mother but by a wealthy widowed aunt in whose house the whole family lived. The patient thought that too much responsibility had been put on her young shoulders; she also felt that, though blamed for omissions, she was never shown any affection or praise for her efforts.

In this setting obedience was made a great virtue, and Anna grew up with a compulsive need for approval and a panicky fear of criticism. The sinfulness of sex had been ingrained in her in earliest childhood by her mother and aunt. During her first admission, a "sex trauma" was interpreted to be of cardinal importance in her abnormal development. At age fourteen she was severely reprimanded for talking to a boy about sex and made to feel that she had committed a carnal sin. This episode was considered the reason for her entering a convent at age eighteen, against the opposition of her father but with the passive acceptance of her mother. Although there were five younger siblings, she claimed she did not know the facts of life and learned about them only in the convent from an older nun who befriended her. In the new evaluation, Anna's entrance into the convent appeared to represent an attempt to retain her mother's approval by devoting her life to a sex-free career. The breakdown occurred when an overdemanding mother superior, with continuous nagging, undermined her own concept of being "the perfect daughter."

This different picture of Anna's early development was reconstructed while she was helping to teach chronically sick children on the pediatric service, an activity that she seemed to enjoy and that was greatly appreciated. Things seemed to be going well until one day a mother told her how much she had helped her little girl and offered to pay her so that Anna would visit her daughter regularly. This praise was too much and made her feel guilty because she "did not do enough." After this she refused to go on with the children's service. She became more restless, was upset about being in the hospital, complained about feeling locked in but was also afraid to go out alone.

Though on the whole she expressed satisfaction with her former work as a teacher, Anna began to express her conflicting feelings about children. She wrote to a friend, "Only I think every child should die instead of trying to live. I don't know the children but I hate to see them get better or even live." As a youngster, in her role as mother's helper, she had been excessively preoccupied with the safety of her younger siblings. When her twin sisters were infants, she was plagued by the fear that the family cat, a placid animal beloved by everyone, might hurt them. She decided to kill the cat, took it with her on a swing, and when she was high up threw it down with all her force. The cat was badly injured and had to be put away. She dated the onset of her fear of animals to this episode. She felt extremely guilty about it, not for killing the cat but for not owning up to it. Following the revival of this memory, she gradually recognized, though with much reluctance, how her excessive "worry" about her siblings, and later about her nieces and nephews, was related to repressed jealousy, dislike, rage, and even hate.

From then on Anna spoke more and more about her "wickedness," the evil within her that could affect other people. Her relationships to other patients changed. In the beginning she spoke of not being worthy of them; now she was afraid she might harm them. A certain competition developed between her and another patient (Zelda, mentioned in Chapter Two), who suffered from a hand-washing compulsion and who was afraid that she might hurt others by transferring germs to them. This was to our ex-nun a crude way of being harmful. Anna could be damaging by her presence alone, by her very wickedness. She feared in particular that she might be harmful to her therapist; if she was immune, then the therapist was "witchy." This fear of doing harm was behind Anna's constant talk of wanting to leave the hospital, of wanting to run. When it was brought up at ward rounds, a senior psychiatrist reminded her that she was here as a voluntary patient and was free to leave. Thereupon she handed in a notice to leave within three days, but then panicked. She accepted the suggestion to retract her notice and to visit her family for a long holiday weekend. In spite of some anxiety she traveled alone and visited a sister and her family.

Anna did not return on the day she was expected but sent a special-delivery letter saying that she had become panicky at the idea of returning to be locked up again; at the same time, she expressed despair about having failed again with treatment. One might have accepted her not returning at face value and thereby terminated treatment. However, it was felt that she was too disturbed and anxiety-ridden to make a rational decision. She was informed in a letter that her leave had been extended: "You may be sure that it is not too late and this is not a failure. I shall expect you back by the end of this week, Sunday at the latest." When she returned, unaccompanied, it was with the definite feeling of having made a voluntary decision.

After this there were marked changes in Anna's attitude toward the hospital. She no longer insisted that every routine was like a convent rule or that every person in authority would ultimately rise to destroy her (her experience with the mother superior). The mother superior had been extremely critical of Anna's teaching methods as too liberal and modern, and severely reprimanded her for being disobedient. Her first symptom of illness had been a severe loss of weight because she felt "unworthy" of eating. Increasingly, fatigue became the leading complaint and she was bedridden for nearly two years. Even at the time of her first admission, the history of her illness, with its many and often changing symptoms, was so complicated that not all the details were recorded. Fatigue continued as a major symptom and "explained" her inability to do anything. She quite openly used it as a weapon to defy every effort to involve her in more active living. Other conspicuous symptoms were trance states when she seemed to be out of touch, at times with hallucinations, loss of smell and taste, claustrophobia and fear of animals, and dramatic choreiform thrashing movements.

After her voluntary return Anna was still capricious and compulsive on the ward, apprehensive and anxious at times, without much initiative; but she began to take part in some of the routine activities. She was much more free and direct in her relationship to her therapist as well as to other physicians, who reported that she talked to them in a friendly way. Then she began to speak of "being different from the way I always was." The main point of this "being different" was that she now wanted to make her own decisions and do things according to her own wishes, not because somebody else expected her to do it. She began to conceive of living without needing the approval of her mother, to whose death she had reacted with increased invalidism and under whose internalized authority she had continued to live. She also lost her fear of being harmful to other patients and became outgoing and friendly. She talked realistically and with lively interest about resuming her career as a teacher.

Three months after admission, treatment was terminated unexpectedly, for financial reasons. Anna left the clinic with sincere regret for not having had a say in this matter, but with the conviction that she had accomplished something. She kept up a rather active correspondence for the first few months and, to everybody's surprise, maintained her improvement. She had become much more independent of her family and was more up-to-date and worldly in behavior and appearance. Anna found a job as a teacher in a somewhat sheltered setting and enjoyed the work. Many years later I received informal follow-up information on her. After a clinical conference in which I had been mentioned by name, a young visiting psychiatrist asked me whether I was the same therapist who had treated his aunt many years ago. Anna had spoken to him, the young doctor, quite often about her long illness and how it had been cured. She had remained well, had married, and he felt that she was leading a satisfactory life.

This brief treatment history reveals several points that seem related to the successful outcome. Quite early an episode occurred that highlighted the central dynamic issue of the patient's difficulties (her refusal to see the medical student). Anna found herself in a bind with deep feelings of guilt about obedience, an interpersonal attitude that her upbringing, and even more the convent experience, had endowed with the highest merit but against which she had secretly rebelled because she felt crushed by it. By pursuing the explanations that she herself offered, other broad issues came to the fore. In particular, her complex symptomatology demonstrated that she had been sacrificed to the needs of others and that her strength had been sapped; thus she had been turned into a complete invalid. She also recognized that if she were to get well, she would lose the position and power of a victim.

This history clearly illustrates how every problem and symptom are significant on various levels and how these patterns are in constant interaction. Anna's refusal to see the medical student expressed a situational problem in the here and now which immediately brought up problems of her early development and previous situations with similar conflict. It was also quite obvious that her behavior expressed something about her concept of the doctor-patient relationship.

Complex patterns of interaction recurred during the treatment period, and each was taken up for clarification. As long as her real feelings remained concealed, Anna felt anxiety and guilt and mistrusted therapy, always afraid that the therapist would turn against her. A second episode of disobedience, her overstaying her leave, was again approached with therapeutic understanding. As she grew more trusting in her attitude toward the therapist, her other relationships became more open. In this setting she could review her development in more realistic terms, and could acknowledge without guilt feelings her desire and capacity for inner independence. The significant point in the ultimate resolution of an illness based on unresolved personality problems is that something occurs in the interaction between patient and therapist which is unlike any past experience. It is the newness of the therapeutic experience which helps in the rediscovery of early paths of development that were abandoned or not permitted to mature.

THE DOCTOR-PATIENT RELATIONSHIP

Patients vary considerably in the way they express their feelings about the therapist and in their readiness to discuss their views of the relationship. Anna was fairly direct in expressing her concern about her therapist's inexperience and trustworthiness, and she became open in communication only after the therapist had been repeatedly tested and found reliable.

Psychiatrists also differ widely in their sense of security and in their need for prestige and personal satisfaction. It is in the nature of being a beginner to feel reassured when a patient expresses special appreciation, but such an admiring relationship is not without its dangers; in Chapter Five I gave an example of psychotic disorganization when treatment was terminated without any exploration of the intense personal feelings involved. Things are usually less drastic, but fostering the dependent status of a patient is nontherapeutic.

Unfortunately it is not only beginners who are obsessed with the need to feel superior in therapeutic skill and who literally live on the unexplored and unchanging dependency needs of their patients. More than anything else, this subtle exploitation of the relationship for one's own reassurance, even self-aggrandizement, is probably the basis for those cases of seemingly interminable therapy. Like an overprotective and possessive parent, such a therapist keeps a patient from moving toward maturity and independence, the legitimate goals of psychotherapy.

Other psychiatrists in their insecurity may expect too much from their patients and superimpose on them their own concepts of how to live or what to do. Or they may exert undue pressure to get confirmation from a patient about their own concept of the patient's troubles, without giving the patient a real chance to express himself. In his disappointment this kind of therapist will become impatient and irritable, beclouding the therapeutic process even more; the patient becomes burdened by the therapist's anxiety instead of finding support in the search for his own needs.

If encouraged and permitted to do so, patients will express their feelings, often in indirect ways but some quite openly. Paul, the schizophrenic young man mentioned in Chapter Four, was quite open in talking about his making a direct study of his therapist, after he had expressed the desire to get well and return to the world. "I'm here looking at you—now you look like yourself, like Dr. B—but then like Abraham Lincoln—that's the honest truth, you look like Abraham Lincoln—happy and sad."

He then recited from the Gettysburg Address and talked of how the Civil War helped to maintain the union. He felt lucky to be in a hospital where he had a doctor who was Abraham Lincoln. He smiled when I commented that apparently he needed some help to emerge a unified person from the civil war within himself.

Soon the relationship between Paul and his therapist became the center of his concern. He wanted to have complete control over me, continuously asked the nurses to call me for extra appointments, and would become angry and combative with my other patients. He expressed his anger and disappointment by changing me from Abraham Lincoln into Adolf Hitler. In such periods all his communication again became delusional. He said repeatedly, "I have never seen a baby born," always adding, "I have never seen a pilot in an airplane." When he was asked if he ever doubted really being the son of the parents who had been so harmful to him, he declared that that was true, he knew he was the son of Abraham Lincoln and a black woman. He became rational, however, when I said that one could well understand how he might wish for a father who would not have permitted the kind of enslavement Paul had suffered from his mother.

This patient's course in the hospital was quite stormy. After he had come out of his catatonic state he was generally friendly and amiable, and gradually became a contributing member of the ward community. However, he was unpredictable and would get into fights whenever he felt the need to prove himself as a man. He finally made a recovery and gained a fairly good understanding of the factors that had contributed to his breakdown. He kept in touch with me for several years and was able to finish his education along the lines of his own interest; he was considering getting married when I last heard from him.

Therapeutic procedure with schizophrenics is far from simple and predictable, even now when psychotropic drugs may help in periods of panic and disorganization. It makes great demands on the innate capacity and resources of the patient, on the skill, patience, and tolerance of the nursing staff, and on the sensitivity, intuitiveness, and personal security of the physician. But there are few experiences more rewarding for a therapist than being a participant in the emergence from the bondage of panic and isolation of a trusting personality willing to take part in life.

THE HOSTILE PATIENT

The therapist's sense of competence and his inner stability are severely tested when he is confronted with expressions of a patient's disappointment or overt hostility. During the process of close reexamination of the patterns of past and current difficulties, emotions, feelings, and attitudes from the past will be mobilized and expressed. As it becomes apparent that things have miscarried not only because of the noxious actions and influences of others, but also because a patient's own responses to people and events reinforced the abnormal direction, a great deal of resentment and other negative emotions come into the open, often with bitter reproaches that the therapist "blames" the patient. It may seem that these negative reactions will interfere with the progress of treatment; actually they are the vital content of therapy and, if one succeeds in clarifying them, a patient will learn to approach life and people in a more spontaneous, efficient, and realistic way.

Though they suffer from their symptoms and painful experiences in relation to other people, most patients feel that their own way of reacting is right and natural, the only plausible way of conducting their lives, and they will react as if they were being criticized or under hostile attack when efforts are made to consider both sides in a disturbing conflict, or when they need to face the extent of their own contribution to their untenable situation.

Motivated by the wish to maintain what they conceive of as the therapist's good opinion, they will resist this kind of inquiry. A patient may feel that the therapist, whom he had tacitly or explicitly expected to be always on his side, suddenly appears to be "against him"—when he confronts him with errors in his own reacting and behaving—and he will confuse the therapist with all the damaging people from his past and respond to him in the same way. The student therapist may feel that he is doing something wrong when a patient rejects his well-meaning efforts and refuses to acknowledge what appears so clear to the therapist. Instead of coming to a better understanding, such a patient, when it is emphasized that he needs to change, will react with outmoded and inappropriate patterns, with petulance, anger, or rage; he may make unreasonable demands for special attention or try to remain in a dependent position. It is these patterns of interacting that make up what are commonly called *transference* and *resistance*. An attentive supervisor can be of great help to a young therapist in recognizing and bringing into the open these negative manifestations, which serve as guideposts to what should be pursued in therapy. But recognizing these reactions as inappropriate does not serve as protection against the onslaught of a patient's unjust attacks and accusations, and a beginner may experience them as a threat to his integrity and as painfully activating his own unresolved conflicts and experiences.

It is particularly difficult to remain objective in the face of hostile attacks when the therapist himself has been unrealistic in his demands on the patient, insensitive to his needs, or preoccupied with his own problems of prestige. Not every expression of anger and hostility on the part of a patient is a "transference" reaction, but it may be, in part at least, a justified response to a therapist's failure to be attentive to the patient's needs, though the particular form of the hostility is determined by the admixture of frustrations and rages accumulated through painful life experiences. The therapist's usefulness lies in his ability to react in an objective, unretaliatory way to such attacks, with calm readiness to explore the sources of the aggressive reaction.

Not all dissatisfaction and anger is expressed in an open way; exploring the indirect expressions may make even greater demands on the therapist. I give as an example the behavior of Dr. W, a middle-aged man who came for therapy because of recurrent depressions. His condescending and sarcastic attitude had led to the deterioration of his professional as well as his personal life, but at no time did he express any personal feelings or make any comments about the therapist, assuming that therapy was a common scientific enterprise. He reported in a quite early interview that since adolescence he had made the greatest effort never to let anyone know what he really felt; it was pointed out to him that this attitude might interfere with treatment, that he needed to be especially alert about being honest, not only telling the truth but the whole truth; he eagerly agreed to this. Nevertheless, communication was characterized by continuous concealment.

When an insistent effort was made to clarify his pervasive sense of mistrust, Dr. W expressed the suspicion that the therapist was Jewish. Not only had his mother warned him that he should "never trust a Jew," but he himself had gone through many experiences that justified this attitude. It became soon apparent that his "confession" had done little to alter the situation; mistrust and resentment continued to be expressed as subtle and not so subtle personal attacks on the therapist. When this was examined later, he said the therapist had offended him by considering him anti-Semitic. Because he was put under pressure to express his true feelings, he felt the therapist had forced him into an impossible bind and was therefore responsible for the expressed anti-Semitic ideas, which reflected his mother's attitude and not his own. He himself took pride in being liberal and open-minded.

In such a case it is essential to focus on the underlying problems and not on the glaring hostility. Such a patient needs to face his deep sense of self-mistrust and fear of inner worthlessness, which make his facade of superior functioning so essential and which he so desperately defends. The surface behavior usually is socially acceptable, even admired, and it is therefore difficult to recognize as an expression of a constant fear of being unmasked and found out as inadequate and insecure. It is only when a patient feels safe and permits himself to be less than perfect that he gradually will be able to work along with the therapist and begin to deal with the underlying anxiety and self-doubt. Invariably one will recognize the destructive presence of envy, which poisons everything, including therapy. It is not the patient's hostility that defeats him but his deep sense of insecurity in the presence of anyone who seems to be doing at all well. If a patient is helped to become alert to his insecurity, then he may no longer need his mask of superiority and can begin to observe some of the actual abilities and gifts he may have lost track of.

SEXUAL PROBLEMS

Most if not all patients who come for psychiatric treatment have sexual difficulties in some form or other. In classical psychoanalysis the emphasis is on exploring the vicissitudes of libidinal development. I have seen many patients in consultation where premature emphasis on a sexual issue, or the implication that sexual problems created the disorder, interfered with the clarification of the significant problems. This is apt to happen when pat, ready-made psychodynamic explanations have long been publicized for certain conditions. In anorexia nervosa, for instance, it used to be a nearly automatic response to search for "oral impregnation" fantasies, instead of looking for weaknesses in the sense of autonomy and personal identity. The outcome of such misdirected emphasis is a therapeutic stalemate. There are patients with whom the inquiry about the sexual component, or about other unconscious reasons for the noneating, has been pursued for years. A simple question such as, "When was the last time you felt really comfortable with yourself?" or "What do you remember as the first thing that happened that made you feel dissatisfied with the way you looked?" usually brings a somewhat startled but then relaxed response of how the patient had never felt confident or had envied others who seemed to have self-confidence, or even a specific situation when he felt that something was amiss. One girl who had become anorexic at the age of sixteen remembered a class in English literature, at least three years earlier, where the verse about being "master of your fate" and "captain of your ship" had distressed her. Until then she had felt comfortable about fulfilling the fate that life and her parents had prepared for her; the idea that she was expected to direct her own life was incomprehensible to her.

Even patients with sexual problems as the leading complaint may not be ready to explore the underlying factors until some other, more basic aspect in their self-awareness has been clarified and corrected. Take the case of Tom, a thirty-year-old man who had refused to make a career decision upon graduation from college because he resented the notion of "fitting into a slot." He spent some time abroad and then enlisted in the army before finally deciding on a scientific career. Though gifted in his field, he did not feel at ease about his status, was always afraid of being taken advantage of and of not being considered adequate.

Tom also felt inhibited and disturbed in his relationships with women. He began dating first as a graduate student, but no lasting relationship developed. He had great charm and a wide range of interests and had no difficulty in meeting many attractive young women, each of whom he would talk about with great enthusiasm, but then he would suddenly break off the relationship. It was difficult to clarify the real issues since Tom misinterpreted the function of treatment. He had experienced the need to make a career decision as "coercive." Similarly he reacted to any effort to clarify his behavior as hostile intrusion. Whenever a question was raised, he would close up completely because he thought the therapist's interest deprived him of "his" idea. He was continuously on the alert to being "influenced" and resented facing anything that might reveal him as "wrong." Since he lived in constant fear of being found wanting, he exercised the most rigid control on anything he said: "I cannot talk—it is like making an enemy of myself to myself." He had grown up with extremely rigid concepts of purity, never shared the jokes of other little boys, and reproached the others with "Don't be vulgar." This was at an early age when such an unchildlike word could only be a repetition of what some grown-up had said.

No real progress was made until there was a change in Tom's concept of the therapeutic goal, when he discovered that the need for corrective reevaluation of his attitudes was not an accusation of wrongdoing. It gradually became clear that there were two elements interfering with his relationship to women. One was the cultural expectation, enforcing his own observations, that any girl he dated would become interested in him as a marriage partner. After his first enthusiasm in finding an attractive and responsive girl, he would begin to become tense and anxious; after asking her for a date, he would become angry that he was now under an obligation to keep it and thought she would expect more. His other problem, about which he was even more anxious, was that a woman would expect a sexual response from him. Even when he found a girl attractive, was aroused by her, and responded appropriately, he was at the same time panicked at the idea that she now would expect sexual fulfillment. He was caught in the double bind of considering his own desire as "vulgar" and being considered unmasculine if he did not engage in the sexual act. It took long and careful work before he finally felt free of his inhibiting childhood indoctrination and could value his own desires.

At times something effective can be accomplished in a few sessions, even in a single consultation. I recall from the time of World War II a young lieutenant who was haunted by the fear of not being able to perform sexually. He came for a consultation during his leave before going overseas, after a disappointing attempt. As an adoloscent he had been too reserved and timid to make advances to girls. Now he felt more secure as a person and was proud that he was engaged to an attractive woman, but he did not dare approach her lest he fail to satisfy her. Our talk shifted to his experiences in the army, particularly as an officer candidate. He had done well on the whole, but in describing details he suddenly stopped and then smiled: he had had difficulties in assuming leadership and giving commands. With that he stood up and said he knew now what the trouble was. He canceled the following appointment and phoned at the end of his leave that things had gone exceedingly well.

WORKING THROUGH

Every beginner is bewildered by and expresses concern over the fact that pointing out or explaining something to a patient does not seem to do any good, even if the patient seemingly understands or agrees that it is so—nothing seems to change. This of course is not only the beginner's problem; the difference is that the more experienced therapist knows that correction of lifelong misunderstandings and misconceptions occurs only gradually, step by step, and that a problem needs to be examined and reexamined from every angle, as it relates to past experiences as well as to present difficulties, before the new knowledge can be assimilated and become what is usually called "insight."

The more actively a patient participates in this process of self-exploration, with increasing competence in correcting deficiencies, the greater the chance that the new insight will become effective in changing his patterns of living. There are many educated people who know all about psychoanalysis and the expected complexes, and they readily learn to apply to themselves whatever is discussed, but it remains intellectual knowledge and seems to have little effect in promoting true understanding.

At times even what appears to be free and open communication may be an expression of a defensive maneuver or a transference attitude, and what looks like fluency may only obscure the issue. As an example I should like to cite the treatment history of Alfred, a twenty-eight-year-old man who was having difficulties in finishing his Ph.D. thesis. He was depressed about this and also about a poor marriage. He had been in treatment before and appeared a promising candidate for psychotherapy. Alfred was articulate, introspective, and appeared eager to come to a better self-understanding. Gradually it became apparent that his very fluency interfered with his efforts. He spoke incessantly in long sentences and grew peeved and upset when he was asked for clarification or even more when he was interrupted. Being listened to seemed an essential experience for him, more important than whether he was understood or not. The therapist was reduced to the role of waiting patiently for him to finish and was not permitted to single out for special attention anything he said. When an effort was made to clarify this misuse of language as a barrier to understanding, Alfred felt "put down" and reproached. He could feel respected only when given enough time to express himself, and he complained of feeling devastated by any comment the therapist might make. He became panicky, frightened that he might never get a chance to speak again. This feeling persisted even after he had become aware of its irrational nature.

The Therapeutic Experience

In Alfred's family, language had been used in a peculiar way. Any open expression of anger or disagreement was discouraged, or actively condemned, and polite verbal maneuvers were of the greatest importance. Even now his mother would exasperate everyone by her endless talk and complex reasoning, and her own mother had been even stronger in her aggressive use of language. Alfred's grandmother was a Quaker by conversion and a "belligerent pacifist"; even as a child he had been puzzled by this contradiction. Sunday dinners had been pleasant, with much interesting table conversation, but they had left him with a false set of values about the power of knowledge. Readiness to expound on any subject and to hold the floor were all-important. Grandmother dominated these conversations and would put everyone in his place with devastating remarks. All members of this family thought that the word was mightier than the sword, and this is where Alfred acquired his insidious and aggressive use of language.

As the therapist was permitted to take part in examining these problems, many indirect points began to emerge. For Alfred any discussion, particularly when there was disagreement, carried the danger that one person would be annihilated. Though he enjoyed persuading people, swaying them with his arguments, he would later become fearful that the others would be hurt by the fact that their arguments had been rejected and would turn against him. He felt constantly caught in unsolvable dilemmas. When alone he felt threatened by the fear of "nonexistence" because there was no confirmation from another person; on the other hand, in the presence of others he was preoccupied with the question of who would survive and who would be extinguished. Anything that he might do successfully, be it at work or elsewhere, implied destroying somebody else, but having nobody around rendered him nonfunctioning. His interaction with the therapist followed a similar pattern. Through his excessive talking he attempted to be in control, but then he became afraid of crushing the therapist and thus depriving himself of the needed help.

Progress with such subtle problems may be discouragingly slow. Many situations and problems need to be clarified over and over until the patient gradually gains an inner conviction that he is regarded with respect, is treated as an existent human being, even when he does not talk but listens to or exchanges views with someone else. It is this gradual transformation—from doubts or outright rejection to intellectual listening and finally to meaningful inner integration—that is covered by the term "working through." This process plays an important role in all therapeutic encounters, though it is particularly drawn-out in obsessive compulsive neurosis and character disorders.

INDICATIONS OF PROGRESS

Patients vary widely in the way they let us know that something useful is taking place. Usually there is some immediate improvement upon the beginning of treatment, in the manifest symptoms and also in mood and general outlook. This is related to the feeling of relief in finding someone who appears truly interested and is willing to listen.

In some there is dramatic improvement, with the patient proudly declaring that all his troubles are settled. Not uncommonly this takes place in those who have been quite doubtful, even aggressively negativistic, about the need for psychiatric help and who will suddenly stop all their complaints and undergo a conversion to health. During my residency I saw Mrs. K, who had become a complete invalid during the preceding seven years because of "polio" she had suffered while traveling with her husband. A severe contraction in one leg kept her from walking and she was in a wheel chair. She came to the hospital for surgical correction, but she was so emotional that the orthopedist requested a psychiatric evaluation. She violently objected to this as "too drastic" and would go into great detail to explain why all her symptoms were the natural outcome of the suffering she had undergone. During this detailed review of her illness, a number of contradictions were clarified and events were put into a new perspective—and the miracle happened that the contracted muscles relaxed and she could walk again. Now she was as uncritically enthusiastic about the value of psychiatry as she had been previously defiant and hostile.

Others after a period of negativistic reluctance suddenly begin to pour out their memories and are overeager to learn from past experiences. The task in such cases is to help them recognize the underlying unresolved problems. Such early improvement is called a transference cure, an expression of hope and gratitude toward a helper who is endowed with special qualities and whom the patient wants to appease. Improvement achieved in a short period may be only transitory; but when accompanied by significant changes in attitude, it may be lasting. The story of the former nun who made decisive steps toward greater independence and autonomy in a three-month treatment period may be looked at in this way.

Others proceed slowly and face the troubling issues with more hesitation, often in a veiled way, and changes occur in small undramatic steps during the extended middle phase of treatment. This requires patient listening by the therapist, with gradual clarification of the confused and contradictory messages. It is important to be alert to signs indicating inner changes, however minute. They must be looked for and then brought to a patient's attention because the awareness of such changes in himself encourages his active participation in the process of self-discovery. This careful listening to subtle signs of progress requires patience from the therapist, but not passivity; on the contrary, he must be firm and consistent in confronting a patient with his misconceptions about himself and in familiarizing him with his own abilities. Such an attitude stands in contrast to what most patients have experienced in the past when they were criticized for their shortcomings by impatient parents, teachers, or peers. With such consistent encouragement to uncover his own resources, a patient will gradually perceive the world as not quite so threatening or frustrating. He will stop looking at it in black or white and not be continuously concerned with doing the right thing or live in fear of being blamed for having been wrong. Gradually he becomes less dependent on the approval or disapproval of others, be they people in the present, including the therapist, or the by now imaginary ghosts of the past. Finally, as he begins looking at himself in realistic terms, with less self-condemnation or dislike, he also develops the courage to assume responsibility for his own life.

This phase of treatment requires great alertness on the part of the therapist: he must know when the patient is expressing something in more independent terms, to which he will tactfully agree, though he must be careful to avoid making himself a new agency of approval of disapproval. Such changes in a patient's attitude may be expressed in the way he views his own development, in particular his family life. At the beginning of treatment he may describe his parents as perfect; then come violent expressions of resentment and hatred toward them for having mistreated him; finally, as he gradually frees himself from his excessive involvement with the parents, he becomes capable of seeing their shortcomings and his specific difficulties with them in a broader perspective. He is no longer obsessed with thoughts of revenge and no longer ready to sacrifice his life to his vindictiveness (his very illness represented a monument to their failure). Not all achieve this final resolution. Unfortunately the popularized concept that the patient learns to say in psychotherapy, "I know I hate my mother," is not mere caricature. All too often treatment is discontinued at this stage, when a therapist or patient may feel that recognizing and expressing the repressed anger represents true liberation from a neurotic involvement with the past.

It is dangerous to make generalized statements, but if I were to single out one problem common to all psychiatric patients, it is that they lack the conviction of being an individual, that their "center of gravity" is not within themselves but is somehow invested in others. The intensity of the experience of not being truly oneself varies widely, of course; it is most pronounced in schizophrenics. To describe the task of therapy in general terms, it is to assist a patient in the development of a center of gravity so that he experiences himself as self-directed and takes pride in being the person he is, free to assert himself and to pursue satisfaction in terms of his own goals of living. Many and changing manifestations of this development toward authenticity can be recognized during the slow period of "working through," and every small step in the right direction needs to be acknowledged. One patient who experienced unusual difficulties in making a commitment to his work and also in forming intimate personal relationships—whenever he made some advance he felt immediately afraid that the other person would dominate him—expressed his new recognition of himself as more competent to lead his own life in this image: "Until now I only looked at my toes, afraid that somebody might step on them. Now I can see the horizon, as if the world had opened up for me."

With such genuine increase in spontaneity and self-directedness, accompanied by improved self-esteem and greater self-confidence, a person will be able to live with less strain and anxiety, develop his capacities as an active participant in life, and enjoy what it has to offer. Successful psychotherapy does not do away with problems of living, but it renders an individual more competent in dealing with them.

TERMINATION

If therapy has been pursued in this direction, with a patient's active participation, then there is usually agreement between patient and therapist on when treatment reaches a meaningful conclusion. Sometimes patients are unwilling to take the final step of acknowledging their ability to lead their lives in a more active way, and then it may be helpful to set a reasonable date for termination. Not uncommonly problems that had been rigidly guarded suddenly become accessible under this pressure of time. On the other hand, some patients want to stop before the therapist feels that the treatment goals have been achieved. There is the danger that a therapist, like an overambitious parent, has superimposed his concepts of what the patient should be like and thus handicaps him in attaining true independence. If there has been symptom relief and the patient has made at least some genuine steps toward better self-understanding and greater inner freedom, not much can be gained by persuading him to continue treatment. It is wiser then to let him see how well he functions on his own, and to be available for continued treatment if the need arises. The reassurance that the therapist will continue to be available is of particular importance for schizophrenics. At times the expression of this availability may not amount to more than an exchange of Christmas greetings, with an occasional letter dealing with some difficulty. A permissive attitude about early interruption of treatment does not apply, of course, to situations where anxiety about what he might have to face, impulsiveness, or a hostile interpretation of the therapist makes the patient want to pull out prematurely. This demands careful analysis of motives and, if necessary, referral to another therapist.

8

The Next Step

During the therapeutic process the beginner therapist himself undergoes marked changes in attitude and personality. When things go well, he will gain in self-confidence and sensitivity to his patient's and his own needs. By guiding another person to a more self-respecting attitude toward his inner rights and possibilities, he too will make steps in the direction of greater maturity.

Though I have enumerated here some of the particular difficulties and dilemmas of the beginner, I wish to point out in conclusion that he also has definite advantages in approaching his patients. Not yet routinized or jaded, he can afford to be open-minded and enthusiastic, and this may make up in many ways for his lack of experience. This accounts for the somewhat startling finding that treatment results by beginners are often surprisingly good. Being new at the game and not committed to a definite theoretical formulation, a beginner can permit himself to respond warmly and with true sympathy to a patient's predicament—which encourages the patient to show his own feelings. By helping a patient take a second look at what has gone on in his life and at what he is doing now that interferes with his human relationships, an objective and sympathetic beginner can be effective in therapy.

These early successes in therapy are of great importance for one's development as a psychotherapist. The reward of seeing an anxiety-ridden individual relax, or a frightened and withdrawn one find his way back to active living, will sustain him through the difficult years of learning and refining his skills. Without positive early experiences of seeing troubled people change and improve through their relationship with him, a beginner may conclude prematurely that psychotherapy is a method of little value. He is apt to become anxious and impatient when progress is not as dramatic or rewarding as he had expected. Others will declare patients with whom they have failed untreatable and recommend an organic method instead.

THERAPY FOR THERAPISTS

Those who are successful and who want to continue this work are confronted with the question of how to increase their skills and competence. The conditions for advanced training opportunities, and the availability of more experienced therapists for assistance, vary greatly, and each individual must work out a plan that suits his personal needs and circumstances. Many raise the question during these learning years whether they need a psychotherapeutic experience for themselves. There is, of course, no general answer. It will depend on an individual's needs, the degree of his personal uncertainty and preoccupation with his problems, and the extent to which they may interfere with his therapeutic effectiveness. It has often been stated that people are attracted to psychiatry by their own needs and that their interest is related to their first-hand acquaintance with anguish, depression, and uncertainty. It is probably correct that, lacking familiarity with what mental distress is about, one would not develop such a lasting interest in exploring the deeper aspects of what disturbs others; nor would he have full empathy with what a patient expresses in his indirect, distorted, or disjointed communication. The difference between therapist and patient is a matter of degree, and so is the difference between learning psychotherapy and undergoing it. In order to function effectively, a therapist must develop an objective ability of not letting his problems interfere, and he must find some realistic resolution for his own conflicts. In spite of large areas of uncertainty, he needs a certain hopefulness and confidence in what he is doing; a facade of naive optimism is not enough, nor do pessimism and cynicism have a place in this work.

I have mentioned before some attitudes or expectations of therapists that might interfere with their therapeutic effectiveness. There are those who find the intense personal involvement more demanding than they had expected, arousing undue anxiety or reactivating old personal conflicts, and this may indicate the need for psychotherapeutic help. Others become involved with their patients in an unprofessional way. Needing the patient's adoration and blind faith to bolster one's self-esteem, or otherwise exploiting the intimacy of the relationship for one's own satisfaction, or an inability to listen to the successes and positive achievements of a patient without envy, are problems that indicate a therapist's need for therapeutic help for himself. Such attitudes will gravely hamper him in listening to his patients or giving them the necessary sympathetic and objective attention. Sometimes a therapist is unaware of such attitudes, and the only hint that something is wrong is that too many patients interrupt therapy prematurely or that he finds too many untreatable.

In others it is the increasing awareness of their personal dissatisfaction or unhappiness that make them take the step to undergo therapy, often only after they have observed that psychotherapy can be effective. Still others, though they suffer from personal problems, feel that these do not interfere with their spontaneity and ability to be an alert participant, and they will become competent psychotherapists without undergoing treatment themselves, or will feel comfortable about postponing the decision. By becoming increasingly aware of their own reactions while doing psychotherapy, usually with the help of sensitive supervision, they develop greater emotional maturity and become relatively free from various conflicts. The danger of a therapist's subtly and unconsciously exploiting the psychological plight of his patients will diminish as he becomes more aware of his own reactions, and he will no longer permit himself to be exploited or dominated by them. It is from the positive experience of being an active participant in the resolution of underlying problems and anxieties that a therapist learns to reduce anxieties in others, and also becomes convinced that human conflicts and feelings *can* be durably modified. Psychotherapy can probably not be done without this conviction that psychic difficulties are capable of resolution through an intimate interpersonal experience.

For some the question of therapy for themselves is intermingled with career plans about whether or not to pursue psychoanalytic training. This becomes a matter of practical decision for those in large training centers and in communities with psychoanalytic institutes. A detailed discussion of the desirability of psychoanalytic training is beyond the scope of this book. It is a decision that should be made in a positive way by those who want to contribute to the special individualistic understanding that psychoanalysis makes possible. As a longed-for dream of being let in on some ultimate secret, it plays an unrealistic role in the thinking of many beginners.

There are many students who, in their search for certainty and in the hope that there are definite answers, feel that psychoanalysis is the only road to go, the only reassurance against feeling there is something special they do not know. A question that pervades much of the older literature—the extent to which psychotherapy is equal to or inferior to psychoanalysis—continues to trouble many, not only the beginner. An unfortunate conviction of a hierarchy of values has developed, and it is still implied in many discussions of the 1970s, though probably not as strongly as at the time of my training in the early 1940s: only psychoanalysis deals with causative factors and thus it is the only method that can be truly curative; psychotherapy at best is only a holding operation, where the therapist gives reassurance or support while the patient is "spinning his wheels." This simply is not true. This is not the place to go into the rather special indications for psychoanalytic therapy. But it must be stated explicitly that psychoanalysis is not a cure-all method for every condition: there are many conditions for which it is counterindicated and where appropriate psychotherapy can be more effective.

It is an unfortunate aspect of present-day training that so often it implies a discontinuous learning experience. The advanced training of psychoanalysis is not offered as a consolidation of earlier teaching but is handled as a beginning, requiring a new commitment and extensive study of the voluminous literature and theoretical debates. One must note with regret that the authoritarian organization of the training institute does not encourage free scientific inquiry; independent exploration is not only unwelcome but is often branded as indicating something unfavorable about the questor. Psychoanalysis has undergone marked changes, but innovations are still not accepted unless they come from members of the inner circle, those who first earned their status by being "true believers."

Increasingly often, gifted and independent-minded young therapists finds ways of obtaining informal training instead of attending institutes. They seek out therapists of their own choosing and turn to experienced teachers for consultation or supervision. The possibilities for such continuous education vary widely, and often it requires inventiveness and a willingness to go out of one's way to make personal informal arrangements.

Doing psychotherapy is basically a lonely business, for it is completely geared to the needs of the other person and requires the suspension of concern about one's own needs and inadequacies. But every therapist, young or old, needs friends and colleagues with whom he can exchange opinions, openly discuss problems, failures, and successes, and share broadening experiences. This kind of learning is important for achieving professional maturity. No matter what the theoretical differences may be, it is helpful to be able to share your concerns and anxieties with others and to have someone else available for consultation in periods of doubt.

SOME BOOKS

Reading also plays an important role in the process of widening one's horizon. I shall mention here only briefly a few books that show in broader perspective how psychotherapy can help disturbed people to realize their individuality. My first suggestion is *The Person* by Theodore Lidz (New York, 1968), which gives a broad survey of the life cycle and guides the reader through the major phases and tasks of the individual's development.

For further reading on meeting a patient and learning from the psychiatric interview, there is Harry Stack Sullivan's *The Psychiatric Interview* (New York, 1954), which tells in great detail how to clarify patterns of living and how to come to a useful understanding of what troubles a patient. A more recent book, Roger MacKinnon's and Robert Michels' *The Psychiatric Interview in Clinical Practice* (Philadelphia, 1971), extends the concept of the interview, beyond its immediate application to psychotherapy, to many other clinical situations.

The Next Step

How to apply psychodynamic principles to the interaction with patients has been spelled out in detail by Frieda Fromm-Reichmann in *Principles of Intensive Psychotherapy* (Chicago, 1950). This was the first attempt to make psychoanalytic insights available and understandable to psychiatrists who had no psychoanalytic training. It was also a courageous effort to integrate classical psychoanalytic views with the then very new conceptions of Harry Stack Sullivan. A later book with the same goal of applying the theories of psychoanalysis to psychotherapy in general is Paul A. Dewald's *Psychotherapy: A Dynamic Approach* (New York, 1971). Allen Wheelis discusses in lucid language the goal of psychotherapy in *How People Change* (New York, 1973).

LAST WORDS

Perhaps even more important than sharing experiences with others and learning from books and conferences is the private self-assessment that goes on continuously within each of us. To the student therapist I would give this advice: allow yourself time after treatment sessions to reflect on what has gone on, and train yourself to remember the sequence of events. Also keep careful notes, on at least a few cases, study and reflect on them from time to time, and determine what they convey now in a context different from the actual session. Just as the recovery of a patient is ultimately an inner experience in which he himself must do the agonizing work of reappraisal, so is the learning of psychotherapy a process in which the student himself must do the active work. The continuous reconstruction and reevaluation of what has gone on between you and your patient are necessary steps toward becoming a skillful therapist who is capable of recognizing a patient's needs in disguises that may not coincide with conventional psychodynamics. Reflection aids you to come to some living awareness of the significance and dynamic meaning of the interchange between you and your patient.

It is through such self-reflection and your increasing awareness of inner changes that you become more sensitive to feeling tones and to expressions of your own apprehensions or interfering thoughts and impulses. In this way you grow more effectively objective about your own role in the therapeutic process.